What Others Are Saying

"This book helped change my life! I knew I needed to make a few changes to keep my blood sugar in a healthy range. I have seen amazing results, and like the low carbohydrate Mediterranean Diet approach. I finally have the information I need. Thank you, *Power Healing Foods*."

— *Connie F., Bedford, NH*

"I have low blood sugar and wasn't sure exactly what to do to prevent my blood sugar from suddenly dropping. I learned a lot from the research and personal experience in this book. It helps to know what to eat, and when, to keep my blood sugar steady. I highly recommend having a copy on hand!"

— *Maria P., Tyngsboro, MA*

"Very easy to read. Well-presented information!"

—*Kathy K., Nashua, NH*

1

POWER
HEALING FOODS

Refresh Your Health and Blood Sugar

Paula Constance

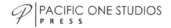
PACIFIC ONE STUDIOS
PRESS

Published by Pacific One Studios Press
www.pacificonestudiospress.com

© 2021, 2022 by Paula Constance

ISBN 978-1-7325349-3-3
1st Edition Revised
Printed in the United States of America

Disclaimer: The information given here is designed to help you make informed decisions about your health and is for informational and entertainment purposes only. It is not intended to replace the advice of a physician or qualified health professional. If you have a condition that requires care, please seek treatment and advice from your health provider. The author and publisher are not medical professionals and are offering ideas and not medical advice. The information in this book is not to be interpreted as a recommendation for a specific treatment plan, product, or course of action.

The publisher and author are not responsible for any specific health or allergy needs that may require medical supervision, and are not liable or responsible to any person or entity with respect to any loss or incidental or consequential damages or negative consequences caused, or alleged to have been caused, directly or indirectly, by the information contained in this book, or for any damages or negative consequences to any person reading or following the information in this book. No warranty may be created or extended by sales representatives or written sales materials.

While best efforts have been used in preparing this book, the author and publisher make no representations or warranties of any kind and assume no liabilities of any kind with respect to the accuracy or completeness of the contents, and specifically disclaim any implied warranties of merchantability or fitness of use for a particular purpose. You should seek the services of a health professional before using any health products or starting any eating, health, diet, exercise, nutrition, or any other program or plan.

Products mentioned in this book are those the author is sharing from personal experience. Any products mentioned are for informational purposes only, and there is no endorsement or recommendation whatsoever by the author or publisher for any food, supplement, or product, or the fitness of any food, supplement, or product to treat any health condition. The information, products, and statements in this book have not been evaluated by the Food and Drug Administration and are not intended to diagnose, treat, cure, or prevent any disease. The author and publisher are not responsible for the choices you make if you decide to use or purchase any of the products mentioned, or products like them. References are provided for informational purposes only and do not constitute an endorsement of any product, brand, or company, or suitability of any product, brand, or company to treat any health condition. Readers should keep in mind that product, health, nutrition, fitness information, and references often change, and some of the information in this book may have changed since it was published.

Trademarks: Pacific One Studios, Pacific One Studios Press, the Pacific One Studios Press logo, and Power Healing Foods are Trademarks of Pacific One Studios, LLC and/or its affiliates in the United States and other countries, and may not be used without permission.

Contents

Acknowledgments

To the many people who made important contributions to this book, you have my sincere thanks and appreciation. A special thank you to Maria, Barbara, and Kathy.

This book is also dedicated to the readers of Power Healing Foods™ who are on a path to refresh their health and blood sugar.

Preface

Growing up, I always had a passion for healthy foods. My uncle lived in New York City when a pharmacist opened one of the first well-known vitamin and health food stores, and he was the first to visit. I have also personally witnessed the powerful and life-changing impact that wholesome foods and nutrients can have on your health.

My healing foods journey started when a family member discovered that she had prediabetes, and was also at risk of low blood sugar. A few weeks later, a close family friend also learned that she had prediabetes. The news was overwhelming. The first thing they wanted to do was find out what foods could change to help lessen their symptoms

It was then that I set out to discover the world's most powerful healing foods and proven natural approaches for healthy blood sugar. The more I researched, the more excited I became to share what I learned about the powerful foods and superfoods that have a remarkable impact on blood sugar, as well as my family's own encouraging journey.

I soon realized this book wasn't only about how to find the best foods and most powerful lifestyle approaches for blood sugar, but it was also about refreshing and nurturing your whole self to live a more vibrant and healthy life. I hope you find a path to good health and refreshment in these pages.

Introduction

I know why you're here. You want to change what the next thirty, or twenty, or even ten years of your life will look like, and you don't want to continue down the path you're on now. The good news is, there is a path of natural healing that can help change all of that.

Why I wrote this book

I understand how you feel. One of my close family members learned that the troubling symptoms she was experiencing—a pounding heartbeat and shakiness—were caused by a spike in blood sugar followed by a dangerously low drop (hypoglycemia). She was sure of one thing: she never wanted to experience those symptoms again. Then a close family friend was upset to learn that her blood sugar was high—she had prediabetes.

When a physician suggested that it was possible to control blood sugar with a change in diet and lifestyle, from that moment forward, I was on a mission to discover the world's most powerful foods and the best natural approaches to support healthy blood sugar.

I have seen firsthand how changing the foods you eat can help keep blood sugar in healthy balance—with remarkable results.

With Power Healing Foods™, you have everything you need to refresh your health and blood sugar—starting now!

How to use this book

Chapters 1-4: What you need to know about prediabetes, low blood sugar, and how to lessen the carb and sugar impact of foods. Also, discover new research about the impact of sleep, how food mindfulness can help, and how to wake up feeling empowered every day to live a healthier and more vibrant life.

Chapter 5: Discover how the glycemic index of foods can help you quickly identify foods that have a high blood sugar impact, and those with hardly any impact at all.

Chapter 6: Find proven and easy to follow eating and lifestyle plans to support healthy blood sugar. Find the best plan for you with your favorite foods!

Chapters 7-15: Why breakfast may be more important than you think, tips to keep blood sugar steady throughout the day, how coffee can help (but not everyone), the truth about artificial and natural sweeteners, organic foods, and more.

Chapters 16-22: In these chapters, you will quickly find the blood sugar impact of almost every food in every food category!

Chapters 23-26: Plan your day with delicious low blood sugar impact breakfast, lunch, and dinner ideas! Also discover power snacks, healthier treats for events and parties, low sugar impact dessert recipes, and more.

Chapter 27: Energizing, delicious and balancing power shakes! Find out what ingredients help the most.

Chapters 28-29: Positive affirmations to get your day off to a great start and a note from the author.

Appendices A and B: Find The 12 Superfoods for Healthy Blood Sugar, a shopping list of my favorite low-sugar-impact foods, and a quick lifestyle checklist.

Chapter 1
Power Healing Foods

Whole foods are healing foods. They provide essential nutrients that help the body balance and heal. They are fresh fruits and vegetables drenched by the sun and nourished by clean, fresh, water. Even the word 'fresh' seems to suggest renewal and healing.

Growing up in New England, my parents told me stories about the fresh fruit they would gather from fruit trees in their yard. I heard about bitter dandelion greens from the garden that would become a healthy salad with savory olive oil and freshly squeezed lemon. I knew about a hidden path that led to shoulder-high wild blueberry bushes providing an unending supply "of the most delicious sweetly-tart blueberries you ever tasted." I heard these stories often, and I knew them all by heart.

I may not have been up at dawn to gather fresh eggs on my great-uncle's farm, or to pick fresh vegetables from his country garden, but I knew the foods they ate were wholesome and rich in healing nutrients.

Vegetables and fruits literally moved from farm to table, and the farm was just outside the window. They didn't use pesticides, herbicides, or artificial sweeteners—and there were very few processed or refined foods. Everything they ate was simple, healthy, and organic—the same foods we now pay premium prices to buy.

It turns out that the path to good health and healing and the healthiest way to live is to not only minimize the amount of refined sugar, pesticides, and chemicals you are exposed to, but to also replenish your body with foods and nutrients that have the power to nourish and heal.

Foods that support healthy blood sugar:

Power healing foods are wholesome foods naturally high in fiber and nutrients that can help keep blood sugar steady. Here are the healthiest foods that support healthy blood sugar, also called power healing foods:

- **Whole grain foods, including oats, barley, and quinoa.** Whole grain foods are high in fiber, B vitamins, niacin, and other essential nutrients. Foods that are naturally high in fiber take longer to digest and are not likely to cause a spike in blood sugar. The natural fiber in whole grain foods also helps slow the absorption of sugar.
- **Healthy protein, including nuts, fish, and unsweetened low-fat yogurt.** Foods like fish, nuts, and unsweetened yogurt, are high in healthy protein that strengthens bones and muscles. Protein also helps slow the absorption of carbohydrates in foods (including sugar).

- **Vegetables, including leafy greens, spinach, tomatoes, beans, and lentils.** Green leafy vegetables, tomatoes, beans, and lentils are a source of essential vitamins and nutrients. These foods are superfoods.
- **Fresh fruits, including apples, strawberries, and blueberries.** Fruits are high in important vitamins, like vitamin C and super healthy antioxidants. Apples and berries are also blood-sugar superfoods that are naturally low in sugar and high in balancing fiber.
- **Healthy fats, including extra virgin olive oil and avocados.** Healthy fats, like those found in olive oil, avocados, nuts, and pumpkin seeds, have a balancing impact on blood sugar. Healthy fats also help slow the absorption of carbohydrates and sugar (a carbohydrate).

The healing power of nutrients

Power healing foods and the nutrients they contain work together to refresh your health and strengthen your body systems. Making empowered food choices can help you take charge of your health—and your blood sugar. The sooner you start, the better you will feel!

Chapter 2
What is Prediabetes? What is Low Blood Sugar?

Study after study shows that a change in diet and lifestyle can refresh your health and help maintain healthy blood sugar.

What is prediabetes?

The foods we eat include protein, carbohydrates, and fats (like olive oil), but the body's main source of energy is from carbohydrates. Carbohydrates eventually break down into sugar (glucose), and glucose provides our cells with the energy they need to function.

If you have prediabetes, your pancreas may have trouble regulating its insulin response to sugar, or your cells may have become resistant to absorbing the sugar they need to function.

When higher than normal levels of unused sugar remain in the blood over time, medical experts explain that it can lead to health problems.

But there's good news! If you have prediabetes, it doesn't automatically mean that you will become diabetic. Studies have found that it's possible for some people to reverse their symptoms and avoid type 2 diabetes with a change in diet and lifestyle.

What changes made the most difference? Eating wholesome foods, reducing fast carbohydrates and foods that are high in sugar, engaging in moderate exercise (like taking a daily walk), and maintaining a healthy body weight.

Blood sugar testing

An (HbA1c) or A1C blood test measures your blood sugar level over the past two to three months.

According to the Mayo Clinic:

An A1C blood sugar level between 5.7% and 6.4% is considered to be in the prediabetes range, while 6.5% or higher, tested on two separate occasions, is considered to be in the diabetic range.

If you test your blood sugar at home, a "fasting" blood sugar level is typically:

- Normal range: Less than 100 mg/dL
- Prediabetes: Between 100 mg/dL 125 mg/dL
- Diabetes: 126 mg/dL or higher (tested on two separate occasions)

Note: A "fasting" blood sugar is taken after you haven't had anything to eat, with only water to drink, for the past eight hours. Your fasting blood sugar is often measured in the morning before a meal.

Blood sugar levels before and after meals

According to the American Diabetes Association (ADA), target blood sugar levels before eating a meal for adults (and women who are not pregnant) are generally:

- 80-130 mg/dL before a meal.
- Less than 180 mg/dL one to two hours after a meal.

Keep in mind, blood sugar levels can change throughout the day depending on what you eat and when. Personal health factors also influence blood sugar levels, so check with your health team to determine your ideal target range.

Note: Exercise, illness, and stress can also have an impact on blood sugar, so if you experience any of these, pay attention to how your blood sugar responds.

Don't get upset over glucose numbers!

The ADA and other diabetes experts remind you not to get upset over your glucose numbers. They are simply a way to see how your diabetes plan is working and if you need to make any adjustments or changes along the way.

Diabetes symptoms

If you are thirsty more than usual, and make more frequent trips to the bathroom, it may be a sign of high blood sugar. Medical experts explain when unused sugar is in the blood, the kidneys try to eliminate it through frequent urination, which can lead to dehydration, making you thirsty to drink more water! Other symptoms of high blood sugar in addition to increased thirst and frequent urination are fatigue, increased hunger, headaches, rapid heartbeat, shortness of breath, unexplained weight loss, and blurry vision.

Keeping blood sugar in a healthy range helps prevent health problems and complications down the road. High levels of unused sugar circulating in the blood over a long period of time may damage the heart or kidneys and lead to neuropathy, among other health problems.

Can high blood sugar give you a headache?

Many things in life can give you a headache, but did you know that a headache may be telling you that your blood sugar is out of the target range? Did you have a meal that was high in carbohydrates? Or eat something with a high amount of added sugar? Pay attention to how you feel after you eat and how your blood sugar responds.

Activities that naturally lower high blood sugar

Moderate exercise, like taking a ten-minute walk after a meal, can help lower blood sugar. How do we know? The America Diabetes Association wrote on diabetes.org: *"exercise can lower your blood sugar up to 24 hours or more after your workout."* A brisk ten-minute daily walk also helped lower blood sugar by 22% in a *Diabetologia* study. Exercise burns energy that is fueled by glucose, naturally lowering blood sugar.

Drinking a glass of water before you exercise can also help lower high blood sugar. Water helps dilute the sugars in the foods you eat, and also helps your body stay hydrated, researchers say.

Hypoglycemia

Hypoglycemia (or low blood sugar) is a sudden drop in blood sugar below the level where your body is able to function (typically below 70 mg/dL). If you have hypoglycemia, and you are not diabetic, your pancreas may have trouble regulating its insulin response to sugar.

If you are diabetic and take medicine, like insulin, you may also be at risk of a sudden drop in blood sugar.

Symptoms of hypoglycemia

The symptoms of low blood sugar (hypoglycemia) include shakiness, a pounding or fast heartbeat, fatigue, excess sweating, weakness, pale skin, hunger, irritability, and feeling lightheaded or dizzy.

A severe drop could result in confusion, disorientation, and loss of consciousness or seizures, warn health experts from the Mayo Clinic.

When is a sudden drop in blood sugar most likely?

According to the Mayo Clinic, a sudden drop in blood sugar is most likely:

- After eating a meal high in carbohydrates or sugar (that may cause your blood sugar to spike, and then drop too low),
- If too much time has passed between meals, after exercising, or
- If you take insulin or other medicines to control diabetes.

Low blood sugar can happen quickly, so pay attention to how you feel and how your body responds.

What to do if your blood sugar drops too low:

If you start to experience low blood sugar symptoms—act fast! The Mayo Clinic recommends having a small portion of fast acting sugar, like drinking a half cup of orange juice, to bring your blood sugar up to a normal range. Check your blood sugar in fifteen minutes. If it's still not in a normal range, they recommended having a small portion of a fast acting sugar.

When your blood sugar returns to a normal range you should start to feel better.

Foods that quickly raise blood sugar:

- A small cup of juice, like orange juice
- A teaspoon of jam, jelly, or honey
- Dried fruit, like raisins (6 to 8 pieces)

Follow with a protein-rich snack

Once your blood sugar returns to a normal range, eating a healthy protein snack can help stabilize your blood sugar, experts from the Mayo Foundation for Medical Research said in an online report. Examples of protein-rich snacks are:

- A handful of nuts, like almonds, with a piece of low-fat cheese

- Apple slices with peanut butter or almond butter (without added sugar, sweeteners, or corn syrup)
- Lean turkey with a piece of low-fat cheese
- Unsweetened Greek yogurt with fresh berries

Tip! Protein and healthy fats help slow the absorption of carbohydrates (and sugar).

Call for help!

If you treat low blood sugar symptoms with a fast-acting sugar, and you are not feeling better, or if you experience severe symptoms, such as confusion, blurry vision, slurred speech, or are about to pass out, don't wait! A severe drop in blood sugar left untreated can be life-threatening. Immediately call emergency responders to help bring your blood sugar up to a normal level.

Chapter 3
A Natural Approach

*Foods and nutrients that naturally support
healthy blood sugar*

Natural healing

The foods we eat and the nutrients they provide are essential
to our health and well-being.

In a *Health Values* study, researchers looked at the
impact that foods and nutrients have on health. They found
that the foods we eat influence our growth and development,
and provide the building blocks to support all of our body
systems. They said, knowledge of nutrition is essential to
prevent illness and disease, and that good health is more
than the absence of disease, but includes our "physical, social,
intellectual, emotional, and spiritual well-being."

I couldn't agree more. If you think about it, wellness is
taking care of our "whole self" and feeling empowered every
day to live a healthier and more vibrant life.

Living a healthy and joyful life every day is a gift you
give yourself.

How effective is a change in diet and lifestyle?

That's what researchers wanted to find out in a landmark *New England Journal of Medicine* study. In the three-year study, people with high blood sugar were asked to follow a healthy, blood-sugar-lowering diet with education and nutritional counseling.

Those who followed the healthy eating plan lowered their risk of developing type 2 diabetes by 58%, while those who took the blood-sugar-lowering drug metformin (with education, but without nutritional counseling) only lowered their risk of developing type 2 diabetes by 31% (compared with those who took a placebo pill with inactive ingredients). The researchers concluded that lifestyle changes and treatment with metformin both reduced diabetes, but lifestyle intervention was more effective.

A food-based approach

In a recent widely-reported Newcastle University study, people in the UK who had type 2 diabetes, and who were also overweight, followed an extremely low-calorie medically-supervised diet for eight weeks. The diet provided three nutritious shakes in place of meals (for a total of 600 calories) and non-starchy vegetables (for an additional 200 calories).

After eight weeks, half of the participants who lost 10% or more of their total body weight were able to restore their natural insulin production, putting their type 2 diabetes in remission. Dr. Roy Taylor, lead researcher of the program, said the researchers believed that in some cases, weight loss in overweight individuals helped decrease fat that may slow or interfere with the functioning of the pancreas. Dr. Taylor remarked, "It was astounding to see the pancreas actually wake up and start making insulin normally again." Everything remained normal after going back to eating ordinary foods and avoiding weight regain, he added.

Study participants who continued to follow a healthy diet with nutrition counseling, were still in remission a year later, without medication. Diabetes UK (Diabetes.org.uk) defined remission as achieving blood sugar (A1C) levels below 6.5% without taking type 2 diabetes medications.

Dr. Taylor said the findings could revolutionize the way type 2 diabetes is being treated. While the research is promising, the UK researchers did not advise that people follow an intense low-calorie diet without consulting with their health care provider to find out what he or she recommends.

A Canadian doctor makes a surprising discovery

After a routine health check, a Canadian physician was shocked to discover that he was diabetic. He said in an online interview that he immediately cut back on carbohydrates, sugars, and starches to "buy time" before deciding which diabetes medicine to take. But something unexpected happened. Within several days, he noticed that he felt better.

He continued following a diet eating non-starchy vegetables, healthy protein, and whole grain foods, with very few carbohydrates, sugars or starches. A few weeks later, he said he was "amazed" and "hugely relieved" to discover that his symptoms had disappeared. It didn't mean he was cured, he said, but more than ten years later he continues to live a healthy life without symptoms, and without medication.

The surprising results that he and others like him have experienced are backed by studies suggesting that a change in diet and lifestyle can remarkably improve your health and blood sugar. This is not only empowering—*it can be life-changing.*

How natural healing works

When you reduce the carbohydrate and sugar load your body has to manage, it can improve your health and blood sugar. Within a few days of following an eating plan that supports healthy blood sugar, you should start to feel better.

Best foods for healthy blood sugar

Start by choosing foods that have a low blood sugar impact:

Where to start:

Choose low glycemic, healthy low carb foods:

- Healthy vegetables, such as spinach and broccoli
- Healthy protein, such as beans, fish, yogurt, and nuts
- Healthy fats and oils, such as olive oil
- Naturally low glycemic fruits, such as berries
- Whole grain, high-fiber foods, such as quinoa

Say "no thank you" to

- "Fast" carbohydrates that quickly become sugar, including highly processed foods made with white flour and white sugar
- Sugary foods, like cake, candy, soda, etc.

Choose healthier alternatives for:

- Foods that are high in saturated fat, like fried foods, bacon, etc.

How to lessen the carbohydrate and sugar load:

- Less than half, or not more than 45% of your daily calories should come from carbohydrates.
- Choose foods that support healthy blood sugar and eat balanced portions to lessen the carbohydrate and sugar load.
- Have a reasonable portion Keep in mind that experts say it takes your stomach several minutes after eating to feel full.
- Replace sweets that have high amounts of added sugar with healthier, low blood sugar impact treats, like a few fresh strawberries topped with a dollop of 2% unsweetened Greek yogurt, and slivered almonds with a dash of cinnamon.

And also do this:

- Pair carbohydrates with healthy protein, like unsweetened Greek yogurt.
- Drink plenty of fresh water.
- Stay active to help keep your metabolism and body healthy.

Manage medications

Did you know that some medicines can lead to high blood sugar in some people over time? While others can increase the risk of low blood sugar? In an online article, medical experts explained that many "commonly prescribed" drugs can increase blood sugar, while other medicines can cause low blood sugar. If you take medication, work with your health care provider and medical team to find out how any medicines you take may affect your blood sugar.

Drink water

Water is essential for all of our body systems to function. Researchers say that water plays "an essential role" in almost every cellular process. It also boosts the metabolism and helps cleanse the body of extra sugar and toxins. These are all good reasons to drink enough water to replenish your body with the water it needs!

Get enough rest

Sleep helps the body recharge from the activities, stress, and demands of the day. But researchers have also discovered that sleep also helps regulate your metabolism and blood sugar.

A study published in *The Lancet* found that when healthy young people without diabetes were allowed only four hours of sleep at night for a week, they experienced a "radical shift" in their ability to process glucose. Sleep has such a positive influence on the metabolism that the researchers said it may one day help with the treatment of diabetes.

The amount of sleep for a good night's sleep can vary from person to person, but most studies recommend seven hours or more of sleep at night for your body to get the restorative rest it needs.

A more restful night's sleep

For a more restful night's sleep, try turning off cell phones, computers, and electronic devices with screens an hour before going to sleep. Why? Scientists say that the blue light from electronic devices mimics daylight and has a stimulating effect on your body. Blue light interrupts your natural sleep rhythm when it's time for your body to naturally relax and wind down.

Instead, set this time aside to listen to soothing music, to pray, meditate, or read something calming or uplifting. This will give your body and mind the time it needs to naturally wind down and prepare for a more restful night's sleep. You may not notice an immediate difference—but your body will.

Can taking a nap help?

If you feel sleepy in the afternoon and find your eyes closing, taking a short nap may help.

In an *Endocrine Society Journal of Clinical Endocrinology & Metabolism (JCEM)* study, researchers found when people who had less than seven hours of sleep at night took a 30-minute nap the next day in the early afternoon, it "reversed the detrimental hormonal impact" of a poor night's sleep. If you didn't get enough sleep at night, and feel tired the next day, the study suggests that taking a short nap in the early afternoon may have a positive impact on your health and blood sugar.

Stay active!

Taking a brisk walk for twenty to thirty minutes every day can significantly improve your health, but did you know it can also significantly improve blood sugar? In a recent study, people who walked or participated in moderate exercise for twenty minutes every day for at least five days a week had significantly better blood sugar levels compared with those who did not exercise daily.

Even if you don't walk every day, just getting up to stretch every twenty minutes can also boost your metabolism and help regulate blood sugar, another study found. So, if you find yourself sitting for more than twenty minutes, find a reason to get up, stretch, and stay active!

Energizing foods and foods that weigh you down

Healthy blood sugar is not just about making a list of foods to eat and foods to avoid. It's about replacing highly processed foods and "fast" carbohydrates that quickly become sugar with healthier foods.

It's also about pairing carbohydrates with protein (like unsweetened Greek yogurt) or a healthy fat (like olive oil) to help slow the absorption of sugar. You will quickly discover what foods weigh you down and what foods make you feel energized and have a positive impact on blood sugar.

Notice how your body responds to foods

Take a moment to notice how your body responds to foods you eat and your activities throughout the day. Knowing how your blood sugar rises and falls before and after you eat can help you know what foods and lifestyle choices are best for your blood sugar.

It gets easier over time

Making a change to your diet and lifestyle takes less effort over time!

A study, published in *The European Journal of Social Psychology*, found that some people were able to change a habit in as little as eighteen days, while for most people, a new habit became automatic and effortless after sixty-six days. Mark your calendar—that's only nine weeks!

A little encouragement goes a long way

Everyone does better when they feel empowered to make a change for the better. Making a few changes to some of the foods you eat isn't something you are giving up— it's something you are gaining. You are partnering with your body to help it function better.

For a little extra motivation, you may want to work with a like-minded health coach, join an online support group, or use a goal-setting program or app to help you keep up the momentum and energy to stay with it and live it.

Studies show that people are more successful achieving a goal when they follow a plan, and have support and encouragement along the way.

Practice food mindfulness

Do you find yourself rushing through a meal? I know I do. Wait. Slow down. And take a moment to practice "food mindfulness." It can have a surprisingly positive impact on your health and blood sugar. Food mindfulness is the practice of being "in the moment" and observing how you feel about foods after you eat.

Food mindfulness can also help you become aware of how different foods impact your blood sugar. How do you feel ten minutes after you eat a meal? Do you feel energized? Nourished? Healthier? Are you satisfied with just the right portion?

Food mindfulness helps you become aware of how the foods you choose impact your health, and can help you identify and manage any upset feelings or frustrations you may have about the foods you eat.

When you become mindful about the foods you eat, you can trust that healthy blood sugar is something you can work with your body to support and manage.

Tip! A growing number of people practice food mindfulness to manage prediabetes and blood sugar. Look online for "food mindfulness and diabetes."

Chapter 4
Helpful Vitamins
and Nutrients

Vitamins and nutrients are essential for good health.
Here are a few vitamins and nutrients that can
have a positive impact on blood sugar.

Vitamin B12

If you have high blood sugar, or problems balancing blood sugar, you may want to ask your medical provider to check your level of vitamin B12. A study published in the *Journal of the American Board of Family Medicine* found that 22% of people who had type 2 diabetes also had low levels of vitamin B12.

Why is vitamin B12 important?

Vitamin B12 is an essential vitamin that helps your body function. It helps create red blood cells, rebuilds nerves, and is important for DNA synthesis, according to the National Institutes of Health (NIH).

Those familiar with vitamin B12 note that a deficiency can develop slowly over time, so it's possible that you may become deficient and not even realize it. The symptoms of a vitamin B12 deficiency are fatigue, anemia, weakness, numbness, tingling in the hands, legs, or feet, problems with balance, and difficulty thinking. The NIH experts added that you may have low levels of vitamin B12 if:

- You follow a vegetarian diet or do not eat enough foods that provide high amounts of vitamin B12.
- Your body isn't absorbing enough vitamin B12 from the foods you eat.
- You take medications that interfere with the absorption of vitamin B12.

Natural sources of vitamin B12

Vitamin B12 is found in meat, fish, milk, cheese, sardines, liver, chicken, and eggs. You will also find vitamin B12 in vitamin-fortified cereal.

What is the recommended amount?

The USDA recommends 2.4 micrograms of vitamin B12 a day for adults, but "no upper limit has been set." Mayo Clinic experts say you can safely take higher doses because your body only absorbs what it needs, and the rest passes through the urine.

Your health care provider can let you know if you have a healthy level of this essential nutrient.

Vitamin C

Vitamin C is a powerful antioxidant known for its ability to fight off colds, boost the immune system, and calm inflammation, which is the leading cause of many chronic diseases. But did you know that vitamin C may also help support healthy blood sugar?

When people with type 2 diabetes took 500 mg of vitamin C twice a day, an Australian study found that they experienced lower blood sugar levels throughout the day, and had fewer blood sugar spikes after meals. Another study found that people with type 2 diabetes who randomly received a daily supplement of 500 mg or 1000 mg of vitamin C a day for six weeks had "a notable decrease in their blood glucose levels."

Natural sources of vitamin C

Our bodies are not able to produce or store vitamin C, so we have to get all of the vitamin C our bodies need every day from natural sources. Foods we eat that are naturally high in vitamin C include spinach, red bell peppers, lemons, apples, oranges, tangerines, and grapefruit.

Many people also take vitamin C to supplement their daily needs. Look for quality brands without fillers or added sugar. Capsules are often easier to digest than hard tablets.

The amount of vitamin C used in the study that had a positive effect on blood sugar was 500 mg twice a day.

41

The daily recommended amount of vitamin C is 65 to 90 mg a day for adults, with an upper limit of about 2,000 mg a day. Too much dietary vitamin C is "unlikely to be harmful," experts from the Mayo Clinic experts said, but megadoses "could result in diarrhea or nausea."

Vitamin D

Researchers from the National Institutes of Health Office of Dietary Supplements said that vitamin D is essential for good bone health. It also helps the body fight off illness, strengthens the immune system, and supports healthy blood sugar.

A study published in *The Journal of Therapeutic Advances in Endocrinology and Metabolism* found that people with healthy levels of vitamin D also had better insulin resistance. The researchers also noted that people who have problems with blood sugar are also at higher risk of having low levels of vitamin D.

Natural sources of vitamin D

Natural sources of vitamin D include fish, cheese, and egg yolks. Cod liver oil is also a natural source of vitamin D. You can also absorb vitamin D from the sun, but the sunscreen we use to protect skin from its harmful rays also limits the amount of vitamin D you can absorb. Also, spending more time inside in the winter, and less time in the sun, limits the amount of vitamin D we can absorb from the sun.

The United States has been adding vitamin D to milk since the 1930s to prevent common bone diseases, like rickets. Vitamin D is added to plant-based milk products, but many people in the world still do not get enough vitamin D. World health experts estimated that as many as *one billion people worldwide* do not receive enough vitamin D in their diet from natural sources.

How much vitamin D?

The recommended U.S. daily amount of vitamin D is 600 IU (International Units) for adults, and 800 IU a day for adults over 70. A recent report by The Institute of Medicine noted that it was safe "to take up to 4,000 IU of vitamin D a day." Before adding vitamin D to your diet, check with your health care provider to find out what he or she recommends.

Magnesium

Magnesium is an essential mineral that supports good health and healthy blood sugar. A study published in Science Direct discovered that 25% to 35% of people who had type 2 diabetes also had low levels of magnesium.

Foods naturally high in magnesium:

Foods that are naturally high in magnesium include avocados, pumpkin seeds, almonds, peanuts, legumes, bananas, spinach and green leafy vegetables, and yogurt.

How much magnesium?

The recommended U.S. daily amount of magnesium is 420 mg a day for men and 320 mg a day for women, according to the NIH Office of Dietary Supplements. The NIH experts added that food helps the body absorb magnesium, so if you take magnesium to supplement your diet, be sure to take it with food or a meal.

Different types of magnesium

There are many different types of magnesium available. Registered dietitian Alison Grewal explained in a Livestrong. com article that chelated magnesium is "best for absorption." She explained, "Chelated magnesium is attached to an amino acid carrier, making it easier for the body to absorb."

Magnesium citrate is another form of magnesium often used for its laxative effect, Grewal said. She added that abdominal discomfort, gas or nausea may occur. But if these or other symptoms become worse, promptly contact your physician.

Note: Magnesium can interact with some medicines. Before adding magnesium, or any new supplement to your diet, check with your health care team and medical provider to find out what is best for you.

Chapter 5
The Power of the Glycemic Index of Foods

*There is power in knowing what foods can raise blood sugar
quickly—and what foods have hardly any impact!*

The glycemic index (GI) helps quickly identify foods that
have a high blood sugar impact—and those with hardly any
impact at all. Researchers from the University of Toronto
developed the glycemic index to measure the impact that
different foods have on blood sugar.

The glycemic index ranges from 0 to 100. Foods with a
zero rating have no impact on blood sugar, while foods close
to 100 almost immediately become sugar.

The Glycemic Index

- Low (0–55)
- Moderate (56–70)
- High (70 or above)

You may want to limit or avoid the following high glycemic
foods. They have a glycemic impact of over 70!

Foods with a GI of 70 or higher:

- Bagels
- Cake
- Cookies
- Donuts
- High-sugar cereal
- Mashed potatoes
- White bread
- White flour
- White sugar
- White rice

Low glycemic foods with a GI of 55 or lower:

- Almonds (and other unsalted nuts)
- Apple slices
- Avocados
- Berries
- Sweet potatoes

The Glycemic Load

The glycemic load (GL) is also good to know. It's an estimate of the *total sugar load* of a food that also takes into account how the carbohydrates in a food impact blood sugar.

The Glycemic Load (overall blood sugar impact) of foods

- Low GL (1–10)
- Medium GL (11–19)
- High GL (20 or higher)

Power of the plus sign

An easy way to think about the glycemic load (GL) of different foods without calculating the numbers is to imagine a plus sign (+) after every food you eat that contains carbohydrates.

For example, if you eat a small bowl of whole grain cereal with a few slices of banana for breakfast, and have a small dish of whole grain pasta that is fairly high in carbohydrates with vegetables for lunch, and the combined carbs add up to a high glycemic load, you may want to limit how many carbs you have for the rest of the day to help keep your blood sugar in a healthy range.

The more aware you become of the impact that carbohydrates (and sugar) have on your blood sugar, the easier it will be to find foods you enjoy eating that can also refresh your health.

Chapter 6
How Many Carbs?
Best Healthy Lifestyle Plans

*Keeping carbohydrates in balance can
help keep blood sugar in balance.*

Healthy carbohydrates

Of all the foods we eat, carbohydrates have the greatest impact on blood sugar. To lessen the impact, replace refined carbs that quickly rush into the bloodstream with blood sugar balancing foods, like vegetable dishes, healthy protein, and a moderate amount of whole-grain carbs, such as whole grain or lentil pasta, whole grain bread, oats, and quinoa.

Low carb and healthy carb blood-sugar balancing diet plans:

Here you will find the most successful and popular low carb and healthy carb eating plans and approaches to support healthy blood sugar. Decide on a plan and approach you are excited about and one that will work best for you. Before starting any new diet or eating plan, be sure to check with your health care provider to see if it's a good choice for you.

A Healthy Carb Diet and Lifestyle
200 - 250 grams of carbs a day

Worldwide health experts say the best way to support healthy blood sugar is to limit carbs to 45%-60% of your daily diet. That's **200 to 250 grams a day** for a 2,000 calorie diet, or about 45 to 60 grams of carbs per meal, with an additional 15 to 30 grams for snacks. A slice of whole grain bread, for example, has about 12 grams of carbs. This proven approach, recommended by U.S. and international health officials, includes a moderate amount of healthy carbs.

The Mediterranean Diet and Lifestyle
125 -150 grams of carbs a day

The low carb Mediterranean diet is another great option. In a recent study, people who followed a low carb Mediterranean Diet achieved healthier blood sugar levels. How did they do it?

One third of their daily calories were from carbohydrates, or about **125 to 150 grams of carbohydrates a day** for a typical 2,000 calorie diet.

Meals included plenty of plant-based foods, like vegetables and vegetable dishes, beans, and lentils. The plan also included low-fat cheese, yogurt, olive oil, lean meat, seafood, whole grains, nuts, and fresh fruit, but no sugary or processed foods.

The Keto Diet and Lifestyle
40 - 60 grams of carbs a day

For quick weight loss and fast blood-sugar results, the very low carb Keto diet is a popular choice. The Keto diet allows 10% of daily calories, or *40 to 60 grams* of carbohydrates a day for a 2,000 calorie diet.

Health experts explain that drastically lowering carbs forces the body to burn fat instead of carbohydrates for the energy it needs to function — a process called "ketosis."

Most calories in a Keto diet are from healthy protein, like lean meat and fish, and non-starchy vegetables, such as kale, spinach, tomatoes, mushrooms, onions, broccoli, cauliflower, and asparagus; and healthy fats, such as avocados, nuts, salmon, extra-virgin olive oil, lean meat, cheese, yogurt, and eggs.

Foods higher in carbs that are not part of a very low carb Keto diet, including bread, cereal, grains, pasta, milk, and starchy foods, including most "root" vegetables, such as lentils, potatoes, corn, carrots, beets, peas, and squash.

Desserts that contain sugar (a carb) are not typically part of the Keto diet. Very low carb fruits, including lemons, strawberries, and raspberries, are allowed!

Some people find an extremely low carb diet with limited food choices hard to follow over time, but others say it can achieve quick results.

The Plate Method
Divide your plate!

The American Diabetes Association "Plate Method" is an easy way to balance portions, foods, and carbohydrates without counting carbs! Here's how it works: Draw an imaginary line down the middle of a plate that's about nine inches across, then

- Fill half of your plate with your favorite non-starchy vegetables or vegetable dishes, like salad, broccoli, spinach, or cauliflower.
- Fill one-fourth of your plate with healthy protein, like lentils, chickpeas, fish, lean chicken, or turkey, and
- Fill the remaining section with a whole grain food, like a small piece of whole grain bread or a high-fiber vegetable, such as a steamed sweet potato topped with a small amount of olive oil or dollop of sour cream or unsweetened yogurt—my personal favorite.

Breakfast serving sizes are typically smaller, but the idea is to balance your portions. For example, breakfast could be a scrambled egg with a slice of tomato, a small piece of whole grain toast, and a few fresh apple slices with a sprinkle of cinnamon.

How do the different blood sugar balancing diets compare?

That's what researchers in an *American Journal of Clinical Nutrition* study wanted to find out! They studied the most popular blood-sugar balancing diets to see what approach worked best overall.

Researchers compared The Mediterranean Diet with vegetarian, vegan, low carbohydrate, and low glycemic diets. The researchers found that those who followed the Mediterranean diet had the most significant improvements in glucose metabolism and heart health.

To follow the Mediterranean diet in the study:

- Include plenty of healthy vegetables
- A moderate amount of healthy protein
- Allow about ***150 grams of carbs*** per day for a typical 2000 diet, or 35% of your daily calories

Mediterranean diet foods

- Apples
- Beans
- Berries
- Beets
- Broccoli
- Cauliflower
- Chickpeas

- Cucumbers
- Eggs
- Fish (and shellfish)
- Feta cheese
- Fruits
- Green beans
- Greek yogurt
- Kale
- Leafy greens
- Lean poultry
- Legumes
- Leeks
- Lentils
- Low-fat dairy
- Nuts (almonds, walnuts, flaxseed, etc.)
- Olive oil
- Onions
- Root vegetables
- Seafood
- Spinach
- Squash
- Sweet potatoes
- Tomatoes
- Vegetable dishes
- Whole grains
- Zucchini

Note: The Mediterranean Diet in the study did not include any highly processed foods or foods with added sugar.

A personal story: A small Greek island café

I arrived on the island of Tinos on the last ferry under a canopy of stars. It was after midnight, but I didn't mind. The night was warm, and the hotel was only a short drive from the pier.

With the excitement of being on the island for the first time, I could hardly sleep. The next morning, I was up early looking for a place to have breakfast. I followed a well-kept stone walkway in front of the hotel to a quaint café. The patio had small round tables with white tablecloths shaded by a grapevine-entwined pergola. A flowering pink bougainvillea formed a perfect archway around the entrance.

The proprietor, a sweet older man with a warm smile, waved me over, offering me a choice of seats. The café was open, and I was the first customer.

"Everything looks delicious," I said, looking over the breakfast menu. "What do you recommend?" "Greek yogurt with 'rothakina' (peaches)," he said enthusiastically. It sounded perfect.

In a few minutes, a glass bowl arrived filled with creamy yogurt topped with freshly sliced peaches. I sprinkled a few fresh walnuts on top for a delicious combination of flavors

The owner explained that the peaches were organic and were from an orchard that had been in his family for as long as he could remember.

Leaning back, I wondered what it would be like to have a breakfast like this every morning.

When I learned more about the health benefits of the Mediterranean diet, I thought about my early-morning breakfast. It seemed even healthier under a clear blue sky surrounded by the sparkling Mediterranean Sea. Maybe that was one of the greatest health benefits of all.

Does one approach work for everyone?

I have personally seen good results with the low carb Mediterranean diet and lifestyle. The Mediterranean diet offers a variety of satisfying low carb foods, such as vegetables, avocados, healthy grains, Greek yogurt, olive oil, low-fat cheese, fruit, fish, and nuts. The Divide Your Plate method is also an easy way to help balance carbs and portions.

Researchers say the approach you follow should be based on the foods you enjoy eating, and a lifestyle you are committed to and are excited to follow.

Remember your "why"

A good way to start your day when you get up in the morning is to remember your "why." Why do you want to change your diet and lifestyle for the better? What steps can you take today to make this happen?

Be honest with yourself. What do you need more or less of to achieve your wellness goals? Plan your meals and stay with your plan. If something isn't working for you, make healthy adjustments along the way. Eat foods that support healthy blood sugar that you will enjoy. Participate in moderate exercise every day, eat reasonable portions, and you are already on your way!

Even a small change can make a big difference

If you are overweight, even losing a few extra pounds can improve your health and blood sugar. A study by the National Institutes of Health found that losing only 5% to 7% of your total body weight, or 10 to 14 lbs. for a 200 lb. person, *lowers your risk of developing type 2 diabetes by 58%.*

How to double fat loss

If you want to double fat loss, eat dinner by 6 p.m. In a recent British study, scientists discovered when people ate dinner by 6 p.m., they burned up to 200% more fat in 24 hours than those who *ate the same amount of calories over the same time period* later in the evening.

Another study found that eating dinner later in the evening was linked with weight gain and higher blood sugar levels, even if it was the same meal you would have eaten earlier.

Choose anti-inflammatory foods

It's interesting that many of the foods in a blood-sugar balancing diet are also anti-inflammatory foods. Why is this important? Chronic inflammation has been linked to many chronic health problems, including cancer, heart disease, arthritis, and diabetes, explained health experts from the Cleveland Clinic.

Foods high in saturated fats, like red meat, and highly processed meats, such as hot dogs and bacon, as well as fats like margarine, lard, and fried foods, can cause an inflammatory response in the body over time.

Foods that help fight inflammation include vegetables and food high in unsaturated fats.

Anti-inflammatory foods:

- Fish, like salmon, tuna, and sardines
- Fresh vegetables and leafy greens, like spinach and kale
- Fresh citrus fruits and berries
- Nuts, avocado, and olive oil

Chapter 7
Why Breakfast? Keeping Blood Sugar Steady

Breakfast is the most important meal, but do you know why? You may be surprised by the answer.

Why breakfast?

Breakfast is the most important meal of the day, but it may be even more important than you think.

Researchers from the Cleveland Clinic found when people skipped breakfast, they had blood sugar levels 37% higher than those who ate a healthy breakfast. People who skipped breakfast also had more frequent blood sugar spikes throughout the day, *even when they tried to control their blood sugar by reducing their carbohydrate intake for lunch and dinner.*

What kind of breakfast did the researchers recommend? Eating a balanced breakfast, such as an egg white frittata with vegetables cooked in extra virgin olive oil and a small slice of multigrain toast.

Three-hour rule

To keep blood sugar steady, researchers say to eat small meals throughout the day, and not to let more than three hours go by without having something to eat. Ideally, have a small healthy snack:

Protein-rich snacks:

- A few almonds or walnuts with a small piece of low-fat cheese
- Fresh apple slices with a dab of peanut or almond butter
- A small dish of low-fat cottage cheese or unsweetened yogurt (low-fat) with a few fresh berries
- Hummus with celery sticks

Avoid:

- High carbohydrate snacks
- Sugary snacks

Tip! A small snack between meals can be something simple, like a few almonds or a slice of apple. It can also provide you with an energy boost between meals.

Pair carbohydrates with protein

To help slow the release of sugar, pair a healthy carb with a protein. The reason this works is that protein helps slow the release of sugar, and can help prevent a spike in blood sugar researchers found in an *American Journal of Clinical Nutrition* study. So, the next time you have a meal with a carb, include a healthy protein! For example, if you eat a small slice of multigrain toast (carb), have it with a little olive oil (healthy fat), a small piece of low fat cheese (protein), or almond butter (protein).

For better blood sugar control, save carbs for last!

What happens if you save carbs for the end of a meal? You may have better blood sugar control! A Diabetes Care study found when people ate protein and vegetables, like salad, fish, and broccoli, first, and saved carbohydrates, like whole grains or a slice of whole grain bread, for the end of a meal, *they had significantly better blood-sugar control.* An easy way to remember this healthy eating tip is: *Protein first, carbs last.*

Chapter 8
White Sugar, White Flour, and Fried Foods

Eliminate these foods—and you will be amazed at how quickly you can turn your health around!

"Fast" carbohydrates can quickly rush into the blood stream, overloading your body with more sugar than it can process. Foods made with white flour and high amounts of white sugar are "fast carbs" that quickly rush into the bloodstream.

Here are the most common foods that can cause a rapid rise in blood sugar — *they have a glycemic index over 70!*

Avoid or limit high glycemic impact foods:

- Bagels (instead, choose a small piece of whole grain bread with low-fat cheese)
- Cake, candy, and cookies (instead, choose unsweetened yogurt with berries)
- Cornflakes or puffed rice cereal (instead, choose whole grain cereal topped with fresh berries)
- Macaroni and cheese (instead, choose a small serving of low carb pasta with low-fat shredded cheese)
- Soft drinks (instead, choose unflavored sparkling water with fresh lime, lemon, or orange slices)

- White bread (instead, choose whole grain bread)
- White flour (instead, choose whole grain flour)
- White sugar (instead, choose raw sugar,
  a less-processed natural sweetener, or a
  naturally-derived sugar-free sweetener)

Also, limit fried foods and foods high in saturated fat

Fried foods, and foods that are high in saturated fat, can place a high load on your blood sugar. How do we know? When people replaced foods t *high in saturated fat*, such as hamburgers, bacon, and fatty meats, with foods that were *high in healthy unsaturated fat*, such as vegetables, beans, sunflower seeds, walnuts, and seafood, in a Tufts University study, the participants experienced a *dramatic improvement* in their metabolic health and insulin resistance. The Tufts research showed that eating a diet high in healthy foods and unsaturated fats may help prevent type 2 diabetes.

Good choices:

- Chicken or turkey (lean, grass-fed, ideally organic)
- Fish or shellfish (wild, rather than farm-raised)
- A lean turkey burger, veggie burger, or plant-based burger low in saturated fat
- Dishes made with vegetables, lentils, or beans

A healthier burger

Instead of ordering a beef burger that is high in saturated animal fat, order a plant-based burger or lean turkey burger instead. Add your favorite low glycemic toppings, such as onions, tomatoes, mushrooms, low-fat cheese, or avocado slices. Mustard is a great topping. Look for brands without added sugar. If you add ketchup, read labels. Ketchup may have added sugar or corn syrup.

Choose an "open-faced sandwich" on half of a whole grain roll rather than a full roll — or eliminate the roll entirely — to help lessen the blood sugar and carb impact. Instead of French fries, substitute baked sweet potato fries or a vegetable side dish, like roasted cauliflower. Enjoy a pickle (ideally, without added sugar or high-fructose corn syrup).

You have just transformed a meal that was high in saturated fat into a satisfying meal that is healthier for you, and your blood sugar.

Chapter 9
Artificial and Natural Sweeteners

The surprising truth behind sugar-free and zero-sugar sweeteners—
and what may be a healthier choice.

A personal story: A warning label on gum

"It's not a warning label," my friend announced as we sorted through packs of gum at the checkout counter. "It's a notice. That's what my mom said," he explained. I looked at the package more carefully. It said, "Warning." I wondered why the package had a warning notice. We were both ten years old at the time and didn't give it more thought. We chose a flavor and checked out so we could get to more important things, like playing baseball

It was the first time I remember reading a label and wondering about the ingredients. Today, I look for environmentally sustainable products and foods made with wholesome ingredients. We only have one Earth and one life. We have to take care of our health, one another, and the world we share.

Not all sweeteners are natural

Products with naturally-derived sweeteners are more popular than artificial sweeteners. Here's why:

Avoid artificial sweeteners:

Artificial, sugar-free sweeteners, such as saccharin, aspartame, sucralose, neotame, and advantame can be used to sweeten sugar-free products from diet soda and sugar-free candy to flavored yogurt. While these sweeteners have a sweet taste—some up to 20,000 times sweeter than sugar—they are chemically created sweeteners.

Artificial sweeteners may be "sugar free" and "calorie free," but they are also "nature free." Sweeteners derived from chemicals do not have the natural fiber and cell structures your body recognizes, some experts say. Researchers have also pointed out a possible link between artificial sweeteners and serious health problems. Some studies suggest that artificial sweeteners can disrupt how the body uses energy and processes fat which could lead to diabetes and obesity over time, among other health problems.

For these reasons, naturally-derived sugar-free sweeteners, such as stevia, monk fruit, erythritol, and xylitol, are more popular to sweeten sugar-free products. You will often find these non-sugar sweeteners in everything from mints and gum to cookies.

Know the sweetener in "zero sugar" and "sugar-free" products

When a label says "no sugar added" or "zero sugar" in foods like candy, soda, and yogurt, read the label to find out what sweetener has been added.

Good choice. Naturally derived sugar-free sweeteners:

Good choices:

Here are a few popular naturally-derived non-sugar sweeteners that are not likely to cause a sudden rise in blood sugar:

Monk fruit

Monk fruit extract is a naturally-derived sugar-free sweetener that does not cause a significant rise in blood sugar. Monk fruit can be up to 300 times sweeter than sugar, has no calories, no carbohydrates, and has hardly any impact on blood sugar, making it a popular choice. It also doesn't have the after taste that you may find with stevia.

Monk fruit can be used to sweeten everything from coffee and iced tea to lemonade and yogurt. Try products sweetened with monk fruit to see if it's a good non-sugar sweetener for you.

Stevia

Stevia is a plant-derived sugar-free sweetener that has no calories and does not cause a significant rise in blood sugar. It's also up to 200 times sweeter than sugar. Stevia will not raise glucose levels, and some studies suggest that it may also have a blood sugar-lowering effect in some people. Many people find stevia to be a versatile sugar-free sweetener. Look for brands that have a high percentage of natural stevia rather than fillers. You may want to try stevia to see if it is a good sugar substitute for you.

Sugar-free sugar alcohol sweeteners

You may be wondering if popular sugar-free "sugar alcohol" sweeteners are made from sugar or alcohol. The US Food and Drug Administration (FDA) explains that sugar alcohol sweeteners are not "sugar" or "alcohol." These non-sugar sweeteners are called sugar alcohol sweeteners because their cell structure partly resembles sugar and partly resembles alcohol.

Sugar alcohol sweeteners are often derived from natural sources, like fruits and berries, or are modeled after the naturally-occurring sugar alcohols. They have very few calories and do not have a significant impact on blood sugar.

Erythritol and xylitol are the most popular sugar alcohol sweeteners. They are generally well-tolerated compared with other sugar-free sugar alcohol sweeteners such as HSH, maltitol, mannitol, sorbitol, isomalt, and lactitol, that are more likely to cause digestive upset, gas, and bloating, according to the FDA. Because of this, the FDA requires foods containing high amounts of sorbitol or mannitol to include a warning on the packaging to alert consumers that, "Excess consumption may have a laxative effect."

Good choices:

Erythritol

Erythritol has an advantage over other sugar alcohol sweeteners. It does not cause a significant rise in blood sugar and causes less digestive upset than other sugar alcohol sweeteners.

Studies have also found that erythritol may also help fight the bacteria that causes tooth decay, making it a popular choice.

Xylitol

Xylitol is another popular sugar-free sweetener that is also generally well-tolerated and does not cause a significant rise in blood sugar. A study published in the *International Journal of Dentistry* found that xylitol may help fight the bacteria that causes tooth decay, making xylitol is a popular sugar-free sweetener for gum, mints, and other products.

Xylitol warning for dogs: Xylitol may be well-tolerated in people, but the FDA warns that Xylitol is *extremely toxic* for dogs. In 2014, The American Society for the Prevention of Cruelty to Animals® (ASPCA) Poison Control Center reported over 3,700 xylitol related emergency calls — a dramatic increase over the previous year.

Those familiar with pet health say that xylitol may have a similar toxic effect on other pets, so to be safe, keep all products containing xylitol away from dogs and other pets. Even a small piece of a cookie containing xylitol can be life-threatening. Xylitol can be found in sugar-free gum, mints, cookies, candy, and even peanut butter.

You may be wondering if erythritol is safe for pets. A peer-reviewed report published in *Regulatory Toxicology and Pharmacology* reported that erythritol was not thought to be toxic for dogs, but it may cause digestive upset or other problems. Veterinarian's say, as a general rule, keep all sugar-free sweeteners you are uncertain of away from your pets.

Natural sweeteners:

Below, you will find the blood sugar impact of popular natural sweeteners:

Good choice:

Vanilla extract

Vanilla extract has a very low carb impact and does not cause a significant rise in blood sugar. According to USDA nutrition facts, a tablespoon of vanilla extract only has 1.6 grams of sugar.

When you buy vanilla extract, look for pure vanilla extract made from natural vanilla beans with 35% alcohol. Why? Alcohol is used to naturally extract vanilla from the beans. When vanilla is extracted using alcohol, it also preserves the unique and complex qualities of the vanilla bean, Including its delicate taste.

Natural vanilla extract may also have unique antioxidant properties and possible health benefits, noted a study published in the *Journal of Agriculture and Food Chemistry.*

Where does vanilla come from?

Vanilla is made from tiny vanilla beans found in the pods of the vanilla bean orchid—a beautiful flowering vine that was cultivated thousands of years ago by the native people that lived in what is now Mexico and Central America. Today, Mexico and Central America are no longer the largest producers of vanilla bean extract. Madagascar and Indonesia produce most of the world's vanilla, while Tahiti is known for its own unique variety.

The best quality vanilla extract

When you buy vanilla extract, it's important to know what the bottle contains. Regulatory agencies, like the USDA, make sure that the products we buy are safe, and ensure that the label represents what's inside the bottle.

To make sure what you are buying is actually pure vanilla extract, look for vanilla with a label that says "USDA-certified." A USDA-certified label ensures that the vanilla was extracted from natural vanilla beans and not from other sources, like wood pulp. A USDA certified label also means that the vanilla meets U.S. food quality standards.

Avoid vanilla products with added sweeteners like corn syrup, which can lead to insulin resistance and type 2 diabetes, and also avoid vanilla that contains artificial sweeteners.

Moderate impact natural sweeteners. Use in moderation:

Applesauce

Unsweetened applesauce has a glycemic index of 53 making it a moderate impact food (depending on how sweet the apples are). If you decide to use applesauce to sweeten a recipe, look for unsweetened apple sauce with 4 grams (1 teaspoon) of natural sugar or less per serving.

Bananas

Bananas have healthy nutrients, like potassium and magnesium, and are also naturally high in carbohydrates, make them a moderate impact. To lessen the blood-sugar impact, have a few slices of fresh bananas (but not overly ripe), or about 1/3 of a fresh banana. Ideally, pair banana slices with a protein, like peanut butter, to help slow the release of sugar.

Molasses

Molasses is a rich, dark syrup that is the byproduct of extracting sugar from the sugar cane plant. Molasses has a lower sugar impact than refined sugar. It's minimally processed so it retains many of its nutrients and is a good source of iron, magnesium, and potassium.
One study found that in adults without blood sugar problems, a small amount of molasses helped slow the release of sugar.

If you use molasses, have a small portion to lessen the blood sugar impact. Pair with a protein and drink water to help dilute the sugars.

High impact natural sweeteners. Use sparingly:

Honey

Honey is often called a "healthier" sugar because it contains beneficial antioxidants that have anti-inflammatory properties. Honey also has a GI of 55, which is slightly lower than the glycemic impact of sugar (depending on how sweet it is). But honey is also a sweet, highly concentrated sugar that can cause a rapid rise in blood sugar. If you use honey to sweeten a recipe, use a small amount.

Maple syrup

Maple syrup has a moderate GL of around 54. It's also a concentrated sugar that can cause a rapid rise in blood sugar. Some maple syrup products also contain very little actual maple syrup, but are less expensive sugary syrups with maple flavor. Generally, avoid maple syrup.

Instead, top a whole-grain waffle with a small amount of melted butter, cashew butter, or your favorite nut butter spread. Add delicious unsweetened berries and a protein, like a dollop of Greek yogurt or sour cream to help lessen the sugar impact. Sprinkle with cinnamon for a little extra blood-sugar balancing power. (See Chapter 11 for more information on this Important spice.)

Raw sugar

Sugar has a high glycemic impact with a GI of 65. Refined white sugar has about the same glycemic impact as raw sugar, but raw, unrefined sugar may be a better choice because it is minimally processed and retains more of its natural fiber. Like other high-impact sweeteners, if you use natural raw sugar to sweeten a recipe, use it sparingly.

How much added sugar?

If you eat a serving of food that has 4 grams of added sugar, you are eating about a teaspoon of sugar. Ideally, look for foods that contain 4 grams of sugar (1 teaspoon) or less in a serving size.

Recipes with added sugar

To help lessen the blood sugar impact, if a recipe calls for sugar, try using 1/4 cup less than the recipe calls for, and add extra vanilla extract to help sweeten the recipe. Or use a sugar-free substitute, like stevia, a few drops of monk fruit extract, granulated erythritol, or a combination of naturally-derived, sugar-free sweeteners.

For a little extra balancing fiber, try adding a sprinkle of oatmeal or wheat germ to a recipe, and substitute 1/4 cup of regular flour with almond or whole grain flour. Drinking water can also help lessen the sugar impact of the foods you eat. Have a reasonable portion. Top with a few low glycemic berries and add a dollop of unsweetened Greek yogurt or a teaspoon of low-fat sour cream for a little extra balancing protein.

Limit:

Agave nectar or agave syrup

Agave is a low GI sweetener that will not cause a rapid rise in blood sugar, but some experts say you may want to limit agave nectar or agave syrup because it's made up of almost 100% fructose.

Although fructose may not increase insulin in the short term, some studies suggest that it may contribute to insulin resistance and increase the risk of type 2 diabetes.

Avoid or limit: Corn syrup

Corn syrup, also called corn sugar or high fructose corn syrup, is a less expensive sugar sweetener. Although it's naturally derived, it may not be the best choice for blood sugar. According to an article "Avoid the Hidden Dangers of High Fructose Corn Syrup," Dr. Hyman explains that too much high fructose corn syrup in your diet that can lead to insulin resistance, obesity, type 2 diabetes, and high blood pressure.

Chapter 10
Exercise and Alcohol

*How staying active helps maintain
healthy blood sugar*

Exercise

Do you find yourself sitting for long periods? I know I do. If
this happens to you, find a reason to get up and stay active.
Taking a daily twenty-minute walk can help and studies show
that it can improve your blood sugar.

Here are a few helpful guidelines:

- Twenty to thirty minutes of exercise a day, like
  taking a morning walk, has been shown to significantly improve blood sugar in several studies. (But
  don't overdo it on hot and humid days).
- Before you exercise, eat a balanced healthy snack
  with protein to help keep your blood sugar steady.
- Exercise uses energy that causes a natural drop in
  blood sugar, so before exercising, make sure your
  blood sugar is in a healthy range.

Drinking alcohol

An occasional glass of red wine may help lower your risk of heart disease, and most diabetes experts say it's okay to have a small glass of wine or beer with a meal from time to time, but it's important to know that drinking alcohol can also interfere with your liver's insulin response to sugar.

Drinking alcohol may cause in an increase in blood sugar, followed by an unexpected drop (hypoglycemia). Many of the symptoms of hypoglycemia, like drowsiness, confusion, and difficulty walking, are also symptoms of being drunk, so it may be hard to tell the difference.

If you plan to enjoy an occasional drink with a meal, here are a few tips blood sugar experts recommend to help lessen the impact:

- Before having a drink, make sure your blood sugar is in a healthy range
- Eat a healthy, balanced meal
- Never drink on an empty stomach
- Choose a light drink, such as light beer or a wine spritzer with club soda
- Avoid sugary mixed drinks
- Have a small serving
- Drink water to stay hydrated

Chapter 11
The Balancing Power of
Cinnamon

*This exotic spice was traded three thousand years
ago along ancient shipping routes. Researchers now say
this spice may have more to offer than flavor.*

The balancing power of cinnamon

Sri Lanka is known for palm-tree dotted beaches and tropical
rain forests. It's also the perfect climate for cinnamon trees.

The cinnamon trees in Sri Lanka produce Ceylon
cinnamon that is harvested from the soft inner bark of the
tree. This unique cinnamon is also called "true cinnamon."
Ceylon cinnamon has a peppery cinnamon taste and light
flavor.

The more common Cassia cinnamon, a rich powdery
cinnamon with a stronger taste, comes from the tropical
forests of China, Vietnam, and Burma.

Researchers have recently discovered that cinnamon
may have more to offer than flavor. Studies have found that
cinnamon may have a positive impact on blood sugar. In a
Diabetes Journal study, researchers found when people with
type 2 diabetes added cinnamon to their diet, they had an
improved blood sugar response, without any harmful side

effects. Another study found that daily use of cinnamon may lower fasting blood sugar by up to 29%!

That's a good reason to sprinkle cinnamon on your favorite foods, such as unsweetened yogurt with berries, apple slices, or a whole grain waffle. Use plain cinnamon, without added sugar.

How much cinnamon?

Use Cassia cinnamon in moderation. The powdery cinnamon with a strong flavor naturally contains high amounts of Coumarin, a substance that researchers say may have possible negative health effects in large quantities. To minimize the amount of Coumarin in your diet, limit Cassia cinnamon to "not more than a teaspoon" a day.

Ceylon cinnamon, the lighter, more peppery cinnamon from Sri Lanka, contains only trace amounts of Coumarin, according to a study in *Scientific World Journal*.

Chapter 12
Coffee, Tea, and Caffeine

Coffee can reduce the risk of diabetes in some people,
but caffeine may aggravate symptoms
in others. Here's what to do:

If you enjoy drinking a cup of freshly brewed coffee in the morning, some studies suggested that coffee may help lower your risk of developing type 2 diabetes!

But caffeine may bother some people. Medical experts from the Mayo Clinic noted that in some people, the caffeine in coffee may aggravate their blood sugar symptoms. If you find that drinking coffee aggravates your symptoms, here are a few low-caffeine alternatives:

Coffee

Try drinking naturally (not chemically) decaffeinated coffee and see if this helps. Experts also say to avoid instant coffee. It's more highly processed, so is more likely to impact blood sugar.

If you like coffee drinks, but want to avoid the caffeine and added sugar, instead of ordering a coffee drink made with sugary flavorings and high-caffeine espresso, try ordering a Cafe Ole with steamed "whole milk" and ask for a splash of naturally decaffeinated coffee (instead of high caffeine espresso). For even more blood sugar balancing power, add a sprinkle of cinnamon and a dash of unsweetened dark chocolate powder.

Tea

Tea typically contains less caffeine than coffee, so tea is less likely to aggravate blood sugar symptoms. If the caffeine in tea bothers you, enjoy *naturally* decaffeinated tea, or drink caffeine-free herbal tea.

Benefits of organic tea

There are many benefits to drinking USDA certified organic tea. In an eye-opening investigation by the Canadian Broadcast Corporation, they discovered that many of the popular brands of tea they tested contained trace amounts of pesticides and toxins *that exceeded the allowable limits.*

No one wants to have pesticides or toxins, even in trace amounts, simmering in a delicious cup of tea. To be labeled organic, tea has to be free of harmful chemicals and pesticides. When it's available, organic tea may be a better choice.

Chapter 13
Why Organic?

Organic foods may have greater health and blood sugar benefits than you think! Here's why:

The health advantage of organic foods

Organic foods are among the healthiest foods you can eat. They can't be exposed to toxins or pesticides, they are foods that have not been genetically modified, and are often closest to their natural form, providing more wholesome nutrients.

But before foods can be labeled "organic," they have to meet the following U.S. Department of Agriculture (USDA) quality standards:

USDA standards for organic foods

Foods can only be labeled USDA organic if they:
- Have not been exposed to any prohibited substances for the past three years
- Do not contain artificial preservatives
- Have not been exposed to harmful chemicals, pesticides, or herbicides
- Have not been exposed to synthetic fertilizers

- Have not been genetically modified (GMO) and were not grown from genetically modified seeds

The impact of organic foods on blood sugar

Eating organic, nutrient-rich foods can have a beneficial impact on blood sugar by limiting your exposure to toxins and pesticides, which researchers say, can have a negative impact on the metabolism.

A Science Direct *Environment International* study reported that exposure to pesticides, herbicides, and toxins could disrupt the metabolism and interfere with proper blood sugar and glucose control. For this reason, you may want to include healthy organic foods in your diet when possible.

A personal story: An organic dairy farm

One summer morning, a college friend and I drove through the winding roads of Vermont to visit her family's organic dairy farm. We drove past wildflower fields and quaint New England towns that gave way to sweeping mountain vistas. As we drove, I imagined what it would be like to visit an actual working dairy farm. It turned out to be a weekend I would always remember.

Mornings on the farm began at sunrise. I woke up early and sleepily made my way past the barn to the hillside, where the cows were grazing on a lush green hillside. As I walked closer, I saw more black and white cows than I could count grazing on the hillside.

As I approached, I realized they were much bigger than I thought. I slowly walked up to the closest cow and lightly reached up to pat her side. She curiously turned toward me with a mouthful of fresh grass. I couldn't help but think, *this cow is really is "grass-fed."* She seemed content enjoying the grass and roaming freely among the other cows.

A clanging bell from the main house interrupted my visit. I quickly made my way down the hill and through a large group of free-roaming chickens. They always seemed to be in a hurry, but I was never exactly sure where they were going.

Everyone gathered in the main house for a hearty breakfast. Hot blueberry muffins carried from the oven were placed on a long farm table neatly draped with a red checkered table cloth. They were placed next to bowls of freshly sliced apples, wild blueberries, whole-grain bread and hearty home-made granola. There was also a block of Vermont cheddar cheese, with hard-boiled eggs and a glass pitcher of fresh milk.

But what I loved most about breakfast that morning was that the foods were all farm fresh, organic, and healthy.

Organic dairy

Like other organic foods, dairy products can only be labeled organic when they meet certain USDA quality standards. The standards for USDA organic dairy products include:

USDA Guidelines for organic dairy products:

- Cows can not be exposed to any toxic or harmful substances that can be passed along in the milk.
- Cows can not be treated with antibiotics or artificial growth hormones to produce unnaturally large amounts of milk.
- At least 30% of their diet has to come from grassy pastures where cows can freely graze (often called "grass fed")
- The other 70% of their diet cannot come from feed exposed to chemicals, fertilizer, or pesticides.
- Cows also may not be given feed that contains genetically modified seeds or foods.

This is good news for us—and especially good news for the cows. The healthier cows are, and the more humanely they are treated, the healthier our milk and dairy products will be.

No one wants to consume antibiotics, pesticides, or reproductive hormones in milk or dairy products—even in trace amounts. You may want to choose organic dairy products when possible. It can't hurt—and it may help a great deal.

Chapter 14
Why Non-GMO?

What are GMO and non-GMO foods? Discover the
real risks of genetically modified foods.

What are GMO foods?

Genetically Modified Foods ("GMO," or Genetically Modified Organisms) are controversial because the plants and crops are modified in a lab. Plants or crops are often injected with genetic material from other sources that are not native or natural to the plant, and would not occur in nature.

In the 1990s, genetically modified soybean crops were introduced to farmers by a company that developed a crop that would genetically be resistant to their weed-killing glyphosate herbicide.

This meant that the genetically altered soybean plants could be sprayed with large amounts of the company's herbicide to kill weeds (and any plants that happened to be nearby), but it would not kill the glyphosate-resistant soybean plants. Seeds of the company's soybean plants were sold to farmers, who could then buy and apply more herbicides to kill weeds. Other glyphosate-resistant GMO crops, like corn and cotton, would soon follow.

Should we be concerned?

A growing number of scientists and biologists say we should be extremely concerned about spraying increasingly greater amounts of chemicals and toxins on GMO crops that we consume. Many scientists are also concerned about the impact of introducing large volumes of toxic chemicals into the environment that can run off into nearby streams and lakes, and seep into the soil every year on a global scale.

A study published in the journal *Toxicology* found that exposure to glyphosate herbicides can disrupt the endocrine system and may interfere with the body's ability to regulate blood sugar. Another study published in *Environment Health* discovered that small accumulations of herbicides are starting to show up in people and animals around the world. A recent U.S. Geological Survey National Water Quality Program said that glyphosate herbicides were found in 66 of 70 U.S. streams and rivers near agricultural land.

As for the weeds, there is evidence that they are already starting to adapt to survive. Experts say that glyphosate-resistant weeds are starting to pop up in fields around the world.

Concerns over GMO foods:

- Researchers have no way of knowing how genetically modified foods will be received by the body or if the body receives the same nutritional benefit from genetically modified foods.

- There is no way to tell how your body will respond to unfamiliar cell structures over time.
- There is concern about the unintended long-term impact that genetically altered foods may have on the Earth, the environment, on insects (like honey bees), and on the world's food supply.

How do you know if a food has been genetically modified?

It depends on Federal food labeling laws. If you want to buy non-GMO foods, look for foods that display a "non-GMO" label on their products.

Environmental groups familiar with GMO foods say that at least 70% of soybean and corn crops around the world today are from genetically modified (GMO) plants.

Change for the better

Many scientists and government leaders believe there is an inherently greater value in protecting the foods found in nature—foods that have been nourishing and replenishing the planet we share for thousands of years.

A number of European Union (EU) and other countries have taken the lead by limiting or banning GMO foods. Others are urgently calling for government leaders to strengthen environmental protections. Environmental scientists and lawmakers are also working to limit the use of toxic chemicals by providing economic incentives for companies around the world to create environmentally friendly and sustainable products.

While some say there is little risk in consuming trace amounts of herbicides and other toxins in the foods we eat, advocates of whole foods and healthy living recommend non-GMO foods, fruits, and vegetables.

Many people in communities support local farms and co-ops as a sustainable, earth-friendly choice. To support healthy blood sugar, and overall health, eat wholesome, healthy foods when possible.

Chapter 15
Clean Foods, Safe Packaging

What are 'clean' foods? Everything you need to
know about the healthiest foods you can buy:

What are Clean foods?

In the truest sense of the word, "clean foods" are the healthiest foods you can buy and are the most nourishing foods you can eat. In the Mayo Clinic Speaking of Health blog, nutritionist Eileen Dutter R.D. explained that "clean foods" are minimally processed foods that are closest to their natural form, so "they retain their healthiest qualities and healing nutrients."

Clean foods can be anything from organic berries and vegetables to eggs and yogurt. To find out if the foods you are buying are clean foods, read labels to find out how the food is sourced, processed, handled, and packaged. You will notice the difference. You will also notice how healthy these foods make you feel.

Look for organic foods that are responsibly sourced and packaged from reputable health-minded brands.

Healthy packaging:

Why "BPA-free" packaging?.

Bisphenol A (BPA) is an industrial chemical used to make certain kinds of plastic containers, bottles and packaging. BPA is also sometimes used to make the epoxy lining of cans to protect foods with a long shelf-life from interacting with the metal.

The growing concern is that BPA, and similar chemicals, like BPS, can seep into food and beverages when the plastic containers and packaging containing these chemicals are exposed to heat or acidic foods. This is why it's never a good idea to leave plastic water bottles containing BPA in the hot sun. The heat can cause BPA to seep into the water. When containers containing BPA are used to store acidic foods, like tomato sauce or iced tea with lemon, the acidic content of the food or beverage can also cause BPA to seep into the food or drink from the plastic, researchers say.

Health advocates are concerned about the impact that widespread exposure to BPA, and similar chemicals, has on our health and metabolism. A study published in *The Environmental Working Group* found that BPA acts as a synthetic form of estrogen that has been shown to interfere with how the metabolism and thyroid function. The researchers concluded that increased exposure to BPA may lead to type 2 diabetes and other metabolic problems.

The US Food and Drug Administration allows a certain minimum level of BPA exposure in foods and beverages, but many health-minded companies use BPA free cans and packaging.

To avoid exposure to BPA, BPS, and other chemicals that may be found in plastics, health experts from the Mayo Clinic recommend storing hot foods in glass, porcelain, or stainless-steel containers.

A personal story: Living a BPA-free Life

The vitamin store parking lot in my neighborhood was full on Saturday morning. It happened to be their annual Member's Day event. Tables were set up throughout the store featuring new products. There were samples of delicious low-sugar pecan spice energy bars, dark chocolate protein-powder-covered almonds, and fresh berry protein shakes.

I also noticed a display of perfectly-stacked sports water bottles on a 50%-off table by the cash register. Some were plastic and others were stainless steel. "These bottles are great for outdoor activities," an athletic employee behind the counter said as lingered at the table. I wasn't sure if I needed another water bottle, but I liked the sleek designs. I unscrewed the lid of a wide-rim bottle to look inside. "The plastic bottles are all BPA-free," he said. I was pretty sure I didn't want BPA in my water bottle.

The bottles were well-designed and I liked that they were BPA-free. I decided to buy two; a wide-rimmed BPA-free plastic bottle for traveling, and a stainless-steel bottle with a beach bag clip for the beach.

The more I learned about the metabolic and health risks associated with BPA and other chemicals that could seep into food and drinks from plastic packaging, the happier I was that the sports water bottles I bought were BPA-free.

Chapter 16
Healthy Fruits

*Find out what super-fruits have a balancing effect
on blood sugar, and which fruit juices to avoid.*

Fresh apples are a super-fruit for blood sugar. Other low glycemic impact superfruits include berries and fresh citrus fruits.

You may be surprised that some fruits that have a sweet taste, like peaches, also have natural fiber that can help lower the blood sugar impact.

Recommended serving size

To help lower the impact of the natural sugar in fruits, nutrition experts recommend a serving size of about 1/2 cup of fresh fruit. For very low glycemic fruits, like fresh berries, the serving size can be up to one cup!

Fresh fruits with a low glycemic impact (GI) of 55 or less:

Good choices:

- Apples
- Apricots
- Avocados

- Blackberries
- Blueberries
- Cherries
- Cranberries
- Grapefruit
- Grapes
- Kiwis
- Lemons
- Limes
- Nectarines
- Oranges
- Peaches
- Pears
- Plums
- Raspberries

Apples

Apples are rich in antioxidants, enzymes, and apple pectin—a beneficial, easy-to-digest fiber that also has a stabilizing effect on blood sugar. Apples are also low on the glycemic index with a GI of 39. They also have an amazingly low glycemic load (GL) of 5 due to the balancing effect of apple pectin.

Fresh apple slices are a healthy blood-sugar choice, but you may want to limit applesauce. When apples are processed or mashed into a sauce, they lose a lot of the beneficial natural fiber that helps slow the absorption of sugar. Also, apple sauce may have added fruit juice or sweeteners that can cause a rise in blood sugar. For the greatest health benefit, fresh is best!

Apricots

Fresh apricots are a delicious low glycemic fruit. But fresh apricots bruise easily, so you may have a hard time finding them. Fresh apricots are often found in health food markets and local farm stands, unless you happen to have an apricot tree in your yard.

Dried apricots are a popular snack. They are lower on the glycemic index than other dried fruits and have a slightly lower blood sugar impact, but like other dried fruits, they can be high in concentrated natural sugar. Read labels to see how much natural sugar from the fruit is in a serving size. If you want to have dried apricots, keep the natural sugars to a minimum by having just a few (ideally not more than 4 grams per serving, which equals about 1 teaspoon of sugar). Fresh apricots are a better. choice.

If you decide to have a few dried apricot pieces from time to time, to lessen the sugar impact, have a small portion and pair with healthy protein or fat (like walnuts) to help slow the absorption of sugar.

Avocados

Avocados are rich in flavor, contain healthy nutrients and are high in healthy plant-based fats. They are also naturally high in fiber, have no cholesterol, no sodium, and very few carbohydrates, making them a great low glycemic choice. With a GI under 55, and healthy fats that help slow the absorption of sugar, avocados are considered to be a superfood for blood sugar! Enjoy in moderation, as they are also high in calories.

Blueberries, strawberries, raspberries, and blackberries

Blueberries, strawberries, raspberries, and blackberries are often called blood sugar superfoods. Antioxidant-rich berries have a low blood sugar impact, with GI under 40. They are also naturally high in balancing fiber. The recommended serving size is about a cup of fresh berries!

Cherries

Fresh cherries are known for their powerful anti-inflammatory qualities. With a GI of 22 and GL of around 3, cherries are a great choice, and will not cause a sudden rise in blood sugar.

A study published in the journal *Nutrients* found that cherries also contain potent antioxidants that have anticancer and anti-inflammation properties that can reduce the risk of chronic inflammatory diseases, including arthritis, cardiovascular disease, diabetes, and cancer. The natural fiber in the fruit also helps slow the absorption of sugar. The recommended serving size is about 1/2 cup of fresh cherries.

If you want to use a few dried cherries on a salad, look for brands that are low-sugar or have half the sugar, as most dried fruit can be high in natural or added sugar.

Cranberries

Fresh cranberries are a low glycemic impact fruit. With a GI under 55, cranberries are a good blood sugar choice. Studies also suggest that cranberries contain potent anti-inflammatory antioxidants that have a positive impact on kidney and urinary tract health, among other health benefits.

Recipes made with cranberries and cranberry sauce are often sweetened with sugar because of the tart taste. If cranberry sauce and other recipes with cranberries contain high amounts of added sugar, have a small portion to lessen the blood sugar impact.

What about cranberry juice?

Most fruit juices, like apple juice, pear juice, and orange juice, cause a rapid rise in blood sugar, but low-sugar cranberry juice may be an exception.

A United States Department of Agriculture (USDA) study found that drinking low-sugar cranberry juice may have a beneficial effect on blood sugar. Researchers found that the people in the study who drank a small glass of low-sugar (diet) cranberry juice (with less than 4 grams of sugar per serving) had a lower risk of heart disease and type 2 diabetes. The researchers thought that powerful polyphenol antioxidants in cranberries may have had a regulating effect on blood sugar. Generally, avoid cranberry juice that is high in added sugar or cranberry juice blended with sweet fruit juices, such as pear, apple, or grape juice that can cause a rapid rise in blood sugar. Read labels to find the best low-sugar cranberry juice.

Note: The helpful qualities of cranberries can also be found in cranberry supplements. But check with your doctor and health care team before adding a new supplement to your diet.

Grapefruit and unsweetened grapefruit juice

With a GI of 25 and GL of 3, fresh grapefruit slices are a delicious healthy fruit choice. Grapefruits are rich in powerful antioxidants, vitamin C, and potassium. Fresh grapefruit also has natural fiber in the pulp that helps slow the absorption of sugar.

Unlike other fruit juices, a small serving of grapefruit juice *without added sugar* is not likely to cause a rapid rise in blood sugar, health experts say. One study found that unsweetened grapefruit juice *may even help lower fasting blood sugar in some people.* Fresh grapefruit slices contain natural fruit fiber and are an even better choice.

Tip! Have you ever warmed up a pink grapefruit before eating it? It's delicious. Here's what to do: Cut a grapefruit, like pink grapefruit, in half. Then, separate the natural fruit segments in each half with a knife, being careful not to cut through the bottom of the grapefruit. Place the two grapefruit halves face up on a small flat pan, and broil for a minute or two in an oven (or toaster oven). Watch while heating. It should be warm, but make sure it doesn't burn. Eat with a teaspoon or grapefruit spoon with a serrated edge. Enjoy!

Note: Grapefruit may interact with some medications, so if you take medication, ask your doctor before adding grapefruit to your diet.

Grapes

Although grapes taste sweet, most varieties have a low GI of 53. Grapes also have natural fiber that can bring the GL down to 5, depending on the type of grapes and how sweet they are. Red grapes have an added benefit — they contain resveratrol, a plant polyphenol with super-antioxidant qualities. Studies suggest that resveratrol may have a beneficial effect on heart health *and* blood sugar. The recommended serving size is about ½ cup. Ideally, pair grapes with a healthy protein, and drinking water helps dilute the natural sugars.

Kiwi

Kiwi is a delicious low glycemic fruit with a GI under 53. Kiwi fruit is also high in vitamin A, vitamin C, and natural fiber that can help slow the absorption of sugar.

Lemons and limes

With a GI of 20, lemons and limes are a great fruit choice. Lemons and limes are high in beneficial antioxidants, vitamin C, and natural fiber in the pulp that can help prevent a spike in blood sugar, making them a low glycemic superfood. Lemons and limes can also add a delicious splash of citrus flavor to beverages, soups, and other recipes.

Oranges

Oranges are high in vitamin C, minerals, and potassium. They also have a low GI of around 44, making orange slices a good fruit choice. Fresh oranges also contain natural fiber that can help slow the absorption of carbohydrates (and sugar). But avoid orange juice. When oranges are pressed and processed into juice, they lose their natural fiber, and orange juice will cause a rapid rise in blood sugar. Fresh fruit slices are a better choice.

Peaches, plums, and nectarines

Fresh peaches, plums, nectarines, and other "stone fruits" (fruits that have a pit in the center) are good fruit choices. They have a low-to-moderate GI of 28 to 56, depending on how ripe the fruit is.

Pears

Fresh pears are naturally sweet, and you may wonder if they are high in natural sugars, but they actually have a low GI of 38. The natural fiber in the fruit and skin helps bring the GL down to about 4, depending on how ripe the pairs are. Overly ripe pears will be higher in natural sugars. Generally, avoid overly ripe fruit.

Generally, avoid jarred or canned pears. They are often packed in sweet fruit juice or are high in added sugar. Fresh pears are always the best choice.

High GI fruits with a low-to-moderate blood sugar impact. Have a reasonable portion:

- Bananas
- Cantaloupe
- Pineapple
- Watermelon

Bananas

Bananas contain important beneficial nutrients, like potassium and magnesium, and are below 55 on the Glycemic Index, with a GI of 52, but bananas can have a higher impact on blood sugar, as they are also high in carbohydrates. Bananas moderate Glycemic Load of around 14, depending on how ripe they are. Avoid overly ripe bananas, as they will have higher levels of natural sugar (and a noticeably sweeter taste) and a higher glycemic impact.

To help lessen the blood-sugar impact of bananas, have a few slices, or about 1/3 of a fresh banana that's not overly ripe. Ideally, pair fresh banana slices with a protein, like peanut butter, to help slow the release of sugar.

Cantaloupe

Cantaloupe has a high GI of 65, but it's naturally high in water, bringing the GL down to 4, and making cantaloupe a good fruit choice! Ideally, pair with healthy protein, and have a moderate portion.

Pineapple

Fresh pineapple is high in vitamin C, fiber, and enzymes. Although it has a high GI of about 59, the natural fiber in the fruit brings the GL down to around 7, making it a low-to-moderate impact fruit, depending on how ripe it is.

Generally, avoid overly ripe pineapple, as it will have a higher glycemic impact.

The recommended serving size is not more than 1/2 cup of freshly cut, medium size cubes of fresh pineapple. Drink water to help dilute the natural sugars, and pair with healthy protein, like cottage cheese or unsweetened yogurt, to help lessen the blood sugar impact.

Always avoid jarred or canned pineapple packed in sugary juice or syrup. Also, avoid pineapple juice. Pineapple juice has a high glycemic impact and will cause a rapid rise in blood sugar.

Watermelon

Watermelon is a refreshing summer fruit. It happens to have a GI of 72, but is also naturally high in water and low in carbohydrates, bringing the GL down to around 2! The recommended serving size of fresh watermelon is about 1/2 cup (100 grams), depending on how sweet the fruit is.

Pair watermelon with healthy protein, like feta cheese, to help slow the absorption of sugar.

Moderate-impact fruits

- Dates
- Figs

Fresh dates and figs are moderate-to-high GI fruits, but some studies say that the natural fiber in the fresh fruit can help slow the absorption of sugar.

A recent *Nutrition Journal* study found that eating a small amount of fresh unsweetened dates (of the five varieties in the study) was not likely to cause a rapid rise in blood sugar. Another study found that when people ate fresh unsweetened figs in moderation, they did not cause a rapid rise in blood sugar. They may even have a blood-sugar-lowering effect in some people, the researchers added.

Enjoy a few fresh, unsweetened (but not overly ripe) dates or figs in moderation as part of a balanced diet. Keep in mind that not all foods will impact everyone the same way, so see if fresh dates and figs are a good choice for you.

Limit high-sugar dried fruits

Fresh fruit is always a better choice than dried fruit. When fruit is dried and the water is removed, a high amount of concentrated natural sugar remains, giving dried fruits their sweet taste. Two tablespoons of raisins (or about 1 ounce), for example, have 23 grams of carbs and 18 grams of sugar. That's almost five teaspoons of sugar!

Choose fresh fruit over canned or dried fruit

Try to avoid jarred or canned fruits. They often contain syrup or sweet fruit juices that can cause a rapid rise in blood sugar.

Even packaged unsweetened fruit can contain more than 4 grams (a teaspoon) of sugar per serving! Fresh fruit or unsweetened frozen fruit is a better blood sugar choice.

Choose fresh fruit that is ripe, but not overly ripe. When fruit is overly ripe, the natural sugars in the fruit become more concentrated giving the fruit a sweeter taste, and also increasing the glycemic impact.

Avoid most fruit juice

Almost all fruit juices will immediately cause a rapid rise in blood sugar. Avoid fruit juices like apple juice, orange juice, grape juice, and pear juice. When these fruits are pressed and processed into juice, they lose their natural fiber that helps slow the release of sugar. Many also have added sugar. Except for unsweetened or low-sugar cranberry juice (not blended with other fruit juices), and unsweetened grapefruit juice, avoid all fruit juices, as they will cause a spike in blood sugar.

Note: People taking medications may not be able to drink grapefruit juice, as it can interfere with some medicines.

Pair fresh fruit with healthy protein

To help slow the absorption of the natural sugars in fruit, pair fresh fruit with healthy protein, like unsweetened yogurt, almonds, low-fat cheese, or a dab of peanut, cashew, or almond butter.

Drink water to help dilute the sugars in fruit

Drinking a glass of fresh water when eating fresh fruit can help dilute the natural sugars in the fruit!

A personal story: White tents and fresh apples

On a quiet summer morning, I watched vendors set up a row of white canopy tents in a nearby church parking lot. Trucks of different shapes and sizes lumbered in with fresh produce and other interesting items. A man wearing a casual blazer and white button-down shirt pushed a sign into the grass that said: "Farmer's Market Today." The Farmer's Market was officially open.

The first stand I walked up to had two rows of baskets overflowing with fresh fruits and vegetables.

A pleasant middle-aged woman behind the table carefully placed the last apple on an overly full basket. "These are early apples," she said with a friendly smile.

"They look delicious!" I said, admiring the deep red color with small patches of bright green. A few still had tender green leaves attached to the stems.

Looking over the display of apples, I mentioned I was writing a book about power healing foods and that fresh apples are a "superfood" for blood sugar. "I'm not surprised!" she said, adjusting the baskets. "These were picked this morning. Would you like to try one?"

She offered me an apple from the top of the basket. I thanked her, weighing it in my hand. "It's organic," she added, I think to make me feel better about taking a bite without washing it first.

I polished it on my sleeve until it had a nice shine and took a decisive bite. It was crisp, much juicier than I expected, and surprisingly tart. I also knew that it was loaded with vitamin C, healthy enzymes, and natural apple pectin that is good for healthy blood sugar.

I bought two bags and was happy I stopped by.

Chapter 17
Vegetables, Legumes, and Potatoes

Fresh vegetables are an important part of a healthy lifestyle. Find out what vegetables have little or no glycemic impact.

Enjoy these low glycemic vegetables:

Good choices:

- Artichokes
- Asparagus
- Beans
- Bean sprouts
- Broccoli
- Cabbage
- Cauliflower
- Carrots
- Celery
- Chickpeas
- Coleslaw
- Cucumber
- Eggplant
- Kale

- Leafy greens
- Leeks
- Lettuce
- Lentils
- Mushrooms
- Onions
- Peppers
- Radishes
- Scallions
- Spinach
- Sugar snap peas
- Tomato
- Turnips
- Water chestnuts
- Zucchini

Raw and boiled carrots

Raw carrots are rich in vitamin A and also have natural fiber that helps slow the absorption of sugar. With a GI of 16, raw carrots have a low glycemic impact. Boiled carrots also have a low-to-moderate GI of 32 to 49, making them a good choice.

When carrots are baked, it increases the glycemic impact, so have a small portion. Avoid carrots that are prepared with sugar or sweetened with maple syrup. Instead, season boiled carrots with savory olive oil and delicious spices.

Beans, legumes, lentils, and chickpeas are superfoods for blood sugar!

Beans, legumes, lentils, and chickpeas are superfoods for healthy blood sugar. They are high in nutrients, contain healthy natural fiber, and are low in fat. These superfoods also have no cholesterol and are low on the glycemic index!

A study published in the *Archives of Internal Medicine* found that when people with type 2 diabetes added more lentils, beans, and chickpeas to their diet, they had improved insulin resistance.

Another study in *The Journal of Nutrition* found when people replaced a serving of rice or potatoes with a serving of lentils, it significantly lowered their blood sugar. They also had improved blood sugar levels after eating a meal.

What about "starchy" vegetables?

Vegetables that are high in starch, like white potatoes, are high in carbohydrates that have a high impact on blood sugar. But some vegetables that are high in starches are also high in fiber that can help lower the blood sugar impact. Here are a few examples:

"Starchy" vegetables that have a lower glycemic impact

- Beets
- Butternut squash

- Corn
- Peas
- Pumpkin

Beets

Beets (also called beetroot) have a glycemic index of 61, but the natural fiber in beets brings the glycemic load down to around 5, making them a good vegetable choice. Some studies suggest that beets are also an excellent source of antioxidants that may help support healthy blood sugar.

According to a recent study published in *Nutrition & Metabolism*, powerful antioxidants called phytochemicals found in beets and beet juice may improve insulin resistance and kidney function.

Corn on the cob

Fresh corn on the cob is a gluten-free summer treat. While corn is high in starch that can raise blood sugar, it's also high in beneficial natural fiber that helps lower the glycemic impact.

For example, an ear of corn on the cob, boiled for 15 to 20 minutes, has a GI of about 52, with a GL of about 15, making it a moderate impact food. The natural fiber in corn helps slow the absorption of sugar. Enjoy a half ear of corn at a BBQ or picnic. It's a more reasonable portion that lessens the blood sugar impact.

Most nutrition and diabetes experts say you can enjoy corn on the cob from time to time.

Corn tortilla chips, whole grain

Whole-grain corn tortilla chips contain natural fiber that helps slow the release of sugar, so a reasonable portion of tortilla chips are not likely to cause a rapid rise in blood sugar.

Blue corn tortilla chips have even more whole grain fiber, making them a better choice! Look for baked rather than fried chips. The recommended serving size is about 6 to 8 chips. Add protein, like a dollop of unsweetened yogurt or low-fat sour cream, to help lessen the blood sugar impact. Enjoy!

Pumpkin

Pumpkin has high a GI of 75 but contains natural fiber that brings the GL down to around 3, making it a good choice, when eaten in moderation. To keep the natural sugars down, diabetes experts say to steam, boil, or lightly roast pumpkin. Never added sugar or sweeteners, like brown sugar or maple syrup that can cause a rapid rise in blood sugar.

You can also pair pumpkin with healthy protein to help slow the absorption of sugar. The recommended serving size is typically about ½ cup.

Rutabaga

Rutabaga is a nutrient-rich vegetable that has a high GI of 79, but it's low in carbohydrates bringing the GL down to around 7. Ideally, pair rutabaga with healthy protein. The recommended serving size is about ½ cup.

Sweet potatoes

Sweet potatoes are a superfood for blood sugar! They are high in beneficial fiber and are a good source of vitamin A and potassium. They have a low GI of 44. Studies also suggest that sweet potatoes *may also help achieve better glucose control.*

Ideally, pair sweet potatoes with healthy protein, like a dollop of unsweetened Greek yogurt or sour cream. The recommended serving size is a small sweet potato, baked or broiled.

Limit white potatoes and mashed potatoes

Potatoes are nutritious and are often served with meals. They are naturally high in vitamin C, B6, potassium, and fiber, but they are also high in carbohydrates (starch) making them a high blood sugar impact food. White potatoes are high in starches that can raise blood sugar, and have a GI of 65 to 85 or more.

If you plan to have a baked potato from time to time, eating the skin will help lower the glycemic impact. Adding a dollop of sour cream to unsweetened Greek yogurt may also help. A half potato is a better portion to help lower the glycemic impact.

Mashed potatoes have a high impact on blood sugar. When potatoes are mashed, so is the beneficial natural fiber that could help slow the release of sugar.

Yellow or red potatoes have a slightly lower glycemic impact, according to nutrition experts with the Tufts School of Nutrition and Science. Choose boiled or roasted yellow or red potatoes from time to time. Sweet potatoes are an even better blood sugar choice!

Eating the skin of the potato also provides extra fiber that helps lessen the glycemic impact. Pair potatoes with healthy protein or fat, like fish, olive oil, or a dollop of unsweetened yogurt to help slow the absorption of carbohydrates that can quickly become sugar. Have a reasonable portion as part of a balanced meal.

Chapter 18
Nuts and Seeds

Nuts are rich in healthy protein—and they
may lessen your risk of type 2 diabetes!

A great choice: healthy seeds, nuts, and nut spreads

Seeds, nuts, and nut spreads, like peanut butter, cashew butter, and almond butter, are a high in protein and have no impact on blood sugar. Some studies have shown that nuts and seeds like flaxseeds, almonds, pumpkin seeds, sunflower seeds, macadamia nuts, pistachios, cashews, peanuts, and chia seeds are a great choice for diabetics as they can reduce and help regulate insulin levels. Nuts and seeds are also naturally high in fiber that may also improve blood sugar.

Enjoy a handful of your favorite unsalted seeds or nuts, or use a nut butter spread, like a dab of peanut butter or almond butter on fresh fruit slices, carrots, celery sticks, or whole grain crackers.

Note: Nuts and nut butter spreads are high in protein, fats and fiber, but they are also high in calories, so have a reasonable potion. Unsalted nuts area a healthy choice. Avoid nuts with high amounts of added salt, and nut butters with added sweeteners, like corn syrup, or products that have a high amount of added sugar. *Do not eat nuts or any nut products if you have a nut allergy.*

Good choices:

Nuts and nut butter

- Almonds
- Cashews
- Hazelnuts
- Macadamia Nuts
- Peanuts
- Pecans
- Pistachios
- Walnuts

Seeds

- Chia seeds
- Flaxseeds
- Pumpkin seeds
- Sesame seeds
- Sunflower seeds

Chapter 19
Dairy, Fish, Protein, and Soy

Experts say that protein helps slow the absorption
of carbohydrates, including sugar!

Including healthy protein in your diet is part of a balanced eating plan is an important part of a blood-sugar balancing lifestyle. Foods that are high in protein can help slow the absorption of carbohydrates and sugar.

Good choices:

Fish, shellfish, lean meat, and vegetable protein

- Chicken
- Fish (about two times per week)
- Shellfish
- Tuna (dolphin-safe, low mercury)
- Turkey (free-range, antibiotic-free)

Dairy protein

- Eggs (organic, free-range)
- Cheese (low-fat)
- Milk

- Yogurt (like unsweetened Greek yogurt)

Good to know: Did you know that Greek yogurt contains twice as much protein as other types of yogurt? Also, 1% or 2% unsweetened Greek yogurt contains a higher percentage of protein and fat content that can help slow the release of sugar and carbohydrates. It also has a richer taste!

Dairy milk

Milk is high in protein, calcium, and vitamin D. Dairy milk is also a complete protein that provides the nine essential amino acids your body needs. The protein in milk may also have a balancing effect on blood sugar.

A study published in the *Journal of Dairy Science* discovered when people included milk with their breakfast, the protein in milk had a stabilizing effect on blood sugar. A Swedish study also found that 1% milk may be a better choice than skim milk, as the higher fat content helps slow the absorption of sugar.

According to the USDA, one cup of 1% milk contains about 12 grams of carbohydrates, so be sure to account for this as part of your overall plan. For those who prefer not to have dairy milk, unsweetened almond milk is a popular plant-based milk option.

Almond milk

If you prefer not to have dairy, almond milk is a good choice. A glass of unsweetened almond milk only has only 1 gram of carbohydrates! But almond milk also contains less protein than dairy milk (a glass of almond milk has 1 gram of protein while a glass of dairy milk contains 8 grams).

To add a little extra protein to your diet, have a handful of almonds (about 20 to 30 almonds). a handful of almonds have almost the same amount of protein as a glass of milk! Look for almond milk with vitamin D added, and avoid brands with added sugar or artificial sweeteners.

What about oat milk or rice milk?

Just like the name sounds, oat milk is milk made from oats. People with nut allergies and those who prefer not to have dairy may consider unsweetened oat milk. It's nut-free and creamier than almond milk, but, like other plant-based milk, it's not a complete protein.

Oat milk only contains a small amount of natural fiber. Oats are strained to create oat milk, so the milk has less fiber than super-healthy oatmeal. Look for unsweetened oat milk with vitamin D added. Read the label to decide if oat milk is a good choice for you.

Generally, avoid rice milk as it is often high in carbohydrates that can quickly cause a rise in blood sugar.

Coconut milk

Coconut milk is a plant-based milk made from freshly grated coconut. People sometimes confuse it with coconut water, that is made from the clear liquid in the center of the coconut. Coconut milk that is extracted by pressing the coconut fruit.

Coconut milk is creamy and rich, but coconut milk, and the thicker (and often sweetened) coconut cream, can be high in calories and fat than a plant based milk like almond milk.

Coconut milk is sometimes blended with almond milk to create blended non-dairy milk. If you consider using coconut milk, or adding it to your morning cereal, look for unsweetened coconut milk that is fortified with vitamin D.

The truth about soy and soybeans: GMO or non-GMO?

Soybeans are an important part of the world's food supply. They are also a natural source of plant-based protein. Soybeans used to be grown on rural farms in Japan and across Asia. But today, more than 70% of the world's soybean crops grown and harvested today are genetically modified or GMO soybeans.

The main concern over GMO soybean crops is that they are genetically modified to be resistant to glyphosate weed-killing chemicals, so they can be sprayed with increasingly high amounts of the toxic herbicide to kill the weeds, but not the glyphosate resistant crops.

It's not hard to imagine the possible health and environmental risks of using increasing amounts of weed-killing chemicals on GMO soybean and other crops.

Why limit GMO foods, including GMO soybeans?

Recent studies suggest that glyphosate chemicals, once thought to be safe, are starting to show up in trace amounts in people and animals. Some studies suggest a link between increased exposure to glyphosate herbicides and serious health problems including diabetes, autism, and cancer.

To minimize exposure, even in trace amounts, look for organic, non-GMO soybeans and soybean foods.

Why fermented soybeans are a better choice

Fermented soybeans are a healthier food choice because of the way they are processed, experts say. When soybeans are fermented, they become easier to digest. Researchers say that fermented soybeans may also have possible health benefits.

Good choices:

Fermented soybean products

- Miso soup
- Natto
- Soy sauce

- Tempeh

What about soy and estrogen?

In addition to GMO concerns surrounding soybeans and soy products made using GMP soybeans, researchers have found that soy mimics estrogen.

Studies show that consuming very high amounts of soy and soy products could interfere with your body's estrogen level, metabolism, and thyroid function.

Some experts note that large amounts of soy were used in the estrogen studies, and say that most people should not worry about having a moderate amount of soy in their diet. But others warn against it.

With the controversy surrounding soy and soy products, most nutrition experts say the healthiest option is to choose fermented, non-GMO soy foods, such as natto, low-sodium soy sauce and miso soup. Enjoy, but have a reasonable portion.

Chapter 20
Whole Grains, Pasta, and Ancient Grains

Say 'yes' to quinoa and other whole grain foods.

Whole grain foods are high in beneficial natural fiber that helps slow the absorption of sugar. Whole grain foods are an important part of a healthy, blood-sugar-balancing diet. Have a reasonable serving size.

Most nutritionists recommend a serving size of 1/2 cup of cooked whole grains. It also helps to pair whole grains with a healthy fat (like olive oil) or protein (like unsweetened Greek yogurt or a small dollop of sour cream) to help slow the release of carbs.

Whole grain foods

Whole grain foods, like quinoa, bulgur wheat, and wild rice, are naturally high in fiber and are not likely to cause a sudden rise in blood sugar.

Ancient grains

Ancient grains are the world's original whole grain foods. Ancient grains, like quinoa and spelt, have remained essentially unchanged for hundreds of years.

Whole grains and ancient grains are naturally high in fiber that helps slow the release of sugar.

Good choices

- Barley
- Buckwheat—a non-wheat whole grain*
- Bulgur wheat
- Brown rice*
- Oats*
- Quinoa—a whole grain seed*
- Rye
- Spelt—a unique variety of wheat
- Wild rice*
- Wheat germ
- Whole wheat

*(These grains are also gluten-free)

Bran and wheat germ

Bran is made up of two parts; a nutrient-rich whole grain outer layer, and the wheat germ (or nutritious "heart" of the grain).

Both bran and wheat germ are whole grain foods naturally high in fiber that can have a balancing effect on blood sugar. Bran is also naturally high in nutrients like folate, vitamin E, and thiamin.

Limit

• White rice

Generally, avoid white rice. It's high in carbohydrates that can rapidly become sugar. Brown rice or whole grain rice which takes longer for the body to break down and digest, is a better choice. The recommended serving size is about 1/2 cup of cooked whole grain rice.

Pasta

Whole grain pasta and vegetable pasta (instead of high carb white pasta) are foods you can enjoy in moderation. Whole grain pasta has up to three times more fiber than white pasta making it a better blood sugar choice. Keep your portion size not more than 1/2 cup of cooked pasta to keep carbs in a manageable range.

If you like your pasta cooked lightly, or "al dente," you are already lowering the glycemic impact, diabetes experts say.

Good choices

- Pasta made from lentils or chickpeas
- Pasta made from whole grains
- Pasta made from zucchini or spaghetti squash

Vegetable pastas, like zucchini or spaghetti squash, are "vegetable" noodles that have very few carbs. Pasta noodles made from lentils or chickpeas are also a good choice as they have natural fiber and are low in carbs.

Whole grain pasta is higher in carbs, but has fiber that can help slow the absorption of sugar. All of these choices are than white pasta, which will cause a rise in blood sugar.

The recommended serving size of cooked pasta is generally 1 cup or less.

Limit

- Couscous

Couscous is a very small pasta made from durum wheat semolina. It's also a pasta that is high in carbohydrates, with a GI of 65. If you eat couscous, have a small portion, and ideally pair it with healthy protein to help lessen the impact on blood sugar.

- White pasta

Generally, avoid white pasta. It is high in carbohydrates that can quickly become sugar.

Chapter 21
Bread, Cereal, and Popcorn

*Whole grain bread, cereal, and popcorn can
be part of a blood sugar balancing lifestyle.*

Whole grain foods, like whole grain bread, cereal, and popcorn, are high in fiber and are not likely to cause a sudden
rise in blood sugar. But have a reasonable portion to reduce
the carb impact.

Good choices are whole grain cereal or bread with
a low amount of added sugar—ideally with 4 grams (1 teaspoon) or less per serving. Avoid products made with high
blood sugar impact sweeteners like corn syrup that can rush
into the bloodstream.

Good choices:

- Bran cereal
- Flax cereal
- Granola (without sugar)
- High-fiber cereal
- High-fiber and multi-grain bread
- Nut-based crackers
- Oatmeal and oat cereal
- Popcorn

- Steel cut hot oatmeal
- Wheat and shredded wheat cereal
- Whole grain cereal
- Whole grain crackers

Cold cereal

Toasted oats, bran, shredded wheat, and other whole grain cereals are a good choice and support healthy blood sugar. Ideally, look for cereal with 4 grams (a teaspoon) or less of sugar or less per serving. Avoid highly processed, high-sugar cereals, like cornflakes and puffed rice, that can cause a rapid rise in blood sugar.

Oatmeal

Unsweetened hot oatmeal is a wonderful choice to support healthy blood sugar. Look for rolled (or flattened) oatmeal, or even better, steel cut oatmeal. Steel cut oatmeal is heartier and contains more whole grains than flattened or rolled oats. Both are excellent options. Steel cut oats also come in a "quick cook" variety. Steel cut oatmeal may take a little longer to cook, but the extra wholesome fiber in the oats is worth it.

Instead of adding sugar or sugary syrup, top oatmeal with fresh berries, apple slices, or slivered toasted almonds (protein) with a dash of cinnamon.

Popcorn

Popcorn is a crunchy and satisfying whole grain snack that has a low blood sugar impact. It's also naturally gluten-free!

The healthiest way to prepare popcorn is with a hot-air popper. Add a little butter or salt for flavor, or spritz it with olive oil. For spicy or savory popcorn, try sprinkling popcorn with a small amount of Tabasco sauce, soy sauce, or balsamic vinegar!

If you prefer microwave popcorn, look for the healthiest brand you can find. Some brands of microwave popcorn contain hidden saturated fats, chemical preservatives, or have high amounts of salt or artificial ingredients.

The recommended serving size is a cup or two!

Chapter 22
Healthy Oils and Condiments

What type of olive oil is the healthiest choice? Find out
what experienced olive growers have to say.

Oils are delicious to cook with and drizzle on a salad, but not all oils have the same nutritional value and health benefits.

Highly processed oils lose much of their health benefit and nutritional value when they are highly refined and processed and are exposed to extremely high heat or strong chemicals to extract more oil from the plant, fruit, or seeds. When possible, look for minimally processed, high quality vegetable oils that help slow the absorption of sugar (and carbs).

The most nutritious oils

The most nutritious oils are organic, cold-pressed oils, including olive oil, avocado oil, and sesame oil. These oils are high in healthy fats, nutritional value and flavor.

If a recipe calls for vegetable oil, and you want to avoid highly refined oils, look for minimally processed safflower oil. It's a light, neutral-tasting oil with beneficial fatty acids. A study in *Clinical Nutrition* found that minimally processed safflower oil may also help fight inflammation and have a beneficial impact on blood sugar. Some stores also carry organic, minimally processed canola oil, but it may be hard to find.

Nutritious, minimally processed oils are a great choice to support healthy blood sugar.

Good choices:

- Avocado oil
- Coconut oil*
- Extra virgin olive oil
- Flaxseed oil
- Safflower oil
- Sesame oil

*(Note: Coconut oil is naturally high in plant-based fats, so use a small amount).

The world's healthiest olive oil

Olive oil is popular for a reason. It's delicious and rich in healing nutrients and healthy fats that can help slow the absorption of carbs and sugar.

A study in the *International Journal of Molecular Sciences* found that olive oil may also have beneficial anti-cancer and anti-inflammatory properties.

Organic, extra virgin, first cold pressed olive oil is the healthiest olive oil you can buy. Olive growers explained that "organic" olive oil has not been exposed to pesticides, toxins or harmful substances. "Extra virgin" on the label means that the olive oil has to also meet certain quality standards, including:

- The olives have to be carefully handled and stored.
- Extreme heat or chemical methods cannot be used to process the oil.
- The olive oil has to meet quality flavor standards.

"First cold pressed" oil is extracted from the "first" cold-pressing of freshly harvested olives. Cold-pressed also means that the oil was not extracted using damaging high heat or chemicals.

A personal story: An olive tree in Southern California

One summer, when I visited California with my family, we planned to see a dear friend of my grandparents. She lived on a quiet street just outside of Los Angeles. As we approached the driveway, I noticed that each of the modest homes had a neatly kept yard with an enclosed private patio.

The grandmother greeted us at the door with a big smile and warm welcome. Her husband had passed away several years ago, but she still took great pride in her home. While the coffee was brewing, she led us to the patio to show us her flowers and vegetable garden. It was a beautifully tended garden. The centerpiece was a tall handsome olive tree ripe with olives.

In a charming Greek accent she explained, "My husband and I..." She paused for a moment admiring the tree. "We planted this tree more than fifty years ago... It grew from a tiny sprig." She demonstrated how big a "sprig" was with her thumb and forefinger. I didn't realize you could grow an entire tree from a sprig, but it sounded about right.

"This is the same kind of olive tree that grows in the beautiful seaside village in Greece where I grew up," she added, patting the solid bark like a trusted friend. "I make my own oil from these olives!" She reached up and plucked a few Kalamata olives from the low-hanging branches and handed them to us. I thought, *This tree not only produces delicious olives—it brings her a lifetime of happy memories.*

We gathered around a large dining room table set with her best china. On a colorful ceramic plate, she brought in a large "village salad" for the table. It was overflowing with freshly sliced tomatoes, cucumbers, onions, and green peppers. It was topped with fresh feta cheese, sprinkled with oregano, and generously drizzled with her rich, homemade olive oil. Every ingredient was flavorful and the olive oil had a hearty flavor. But what I liked most, was that it was prepared and made with love.

Chapter 23
Power Breakfasts

Power through your morning with these
nutritious low glycemic foods!

Breakfast is a healthy way to start to your day! Here are a few breakfast ideas that have a low blood sugar impact:

Breakfast ideas:

- Apple peanut butter toast: Whole grain toast (small piece) with peanut butter topped with fresh sliced apple
- Avocado toast with eggs: Toasted whole grain bread with olive oil topped with a scrambled or poached egg, sliced avocado, and a sprinkle of oregano
- Cold cereal, whole grain, high fiber, without added sugar (look for 4 grams of sugar or less per serving). Top with fresh berries and a few slivered almonds.
- Cottage cheese (low fat) with fresh berries, peaches, or pears. Add a sprinkle of whole grain wheat-germ for extra fiber.

- Fresh berries with unsweetened yogurt and toasted slivered almonds
- Scrambled, poached, or hard-boiled egg on whole grain toast with a slice of low-fat cheese and a side of fresh orange slices
- Steel cut oatmeal, without sugar, topped with fresh berries, slivered almonds, and a dash of cinnamon
- Veggie omelet with a small piece of whole grain toast or half of a whole grain English muffin, and a side of sliced tomatoes

Chapter 24
Power Lunches and Dinners

*Satisfying and delicious low carb and
low blood sugar impact lunch and dinner ideas!*

Lunch ideas:

- Chickpea or bean salad
- Fish or shellfish, broiled or baked, with a small side of quinoa or whole grain rice and a vegetable, like broccoli
- Hummus with fresh veggies
- Lentil dish or veggie pasta with stir-fried veggies
- Nuts of all kinds (unsalted) with low-fat cheese and fresh sliced fruit
- Quinoa, brown, or whole grain rice (small portion)
- Salad with fresh mixed greens, tomatoes, cucumbers, radishes, avocado, and sunflower or pumpkin seeds. Add a protein, like a hard-boiled egg.
- Soups, like bean soup, lentil soup, vegetarian and vegetable soup, chicken soup, or minestrone.
- Stir-fry veggies, including asparagus, peas, broccoli, spinach, etc. with a side of quinoa or another whole grain food.

- Tuna salad (Ideally wild tuna, sustainably caught, low mercury.) on butter lettuce with a few whole grain crackers
- Turkey, Swiss cheese, and tomato, open-faced sandwich (low-sodium, free-range, hormone-free) on a small piece of multi-grain bread with no-sugar-added pickles
- Veggie or plant-based burger (low in added sugar and carbohydrates.) Serve with a tomato and cucumber salad or half of a baked sweet potato
- Whole grain taco (vegetarian, chicken, or fish) with salsa (no sugar added or low sugar, not more than 4 grams per serving)

Dinner ideas:

Main dishes

- Bean dishes, legumes, plant-based dishes, and vegetable casseroles
- Fish, like salmon, white fish, and shellfish (wild rather than farm-raised), baked or broiled with lemon and olive oil. (Limit tuna and swordfish, as these are often high in mercury)
- Lean chicken or turkey (free-range, antibiotic-free, and hormone-free)
- Stir-fry vegetable dishes with healthy protein and a side of grains, like quinoa

- Vegetarian dishes
- Vegetable, lentil, and minestrone soup

Side dishes

- Artichokes
- Asparagus with toasted almonds
- Broccoli, cauliflower, or eggplant
- Butternut squash (small portion)
- Green beans
- Lentils, legumes
- Mushrooms, peppers, and onions
- Quinoa, bulgur wheat, and whole grain dishes
- Salad with mixed greens and healthy vegetables
- Spinach
- Sweet potato with skin or yams (boiled or baked)
- Vegetarian chili (without added sugar)
- Wild or whole grain rice (small portion)

Chapter 25
Power Snacks

Enjoy these low glycemic power snacks!

These delicious snacks are not likely to cause a sudden rise in blood sugar!

Low glycemic snacks

- A handful of nuts, such as almonds or walnuts without salt
- Apple slices with a dab of peanut butter
- Avocado and fresh tomato slices drizzled with olive oil and a dash of oregano
- Cauliflower or almond crackers with hummus
- Celery or raw carrot sticks with hummus
- Cherry tomatoes, cut in half, with a dab of olive oil and sprinkle of oregano
- Chicken salad with carrot or celery sticks
- Cottage cheese (ideally low-fat or 1%) with fresh fruit, topped with wheat germ
- Cucumber or celery sticks with unsweetened yogurt
- Hard-boiled egg with fresh veggies

- Tuna salad with a few whole grain crackers (but only occasionally due to the possible mercury in tuna)
- Turkey "roll-up"; Roll a slice of low-fat cheese and low sodium turkey breast together and top with mustard or mayo to create a protein-rich snack.
- Whole grain tortilla chips (6 to 8 chips), especially organic, non-GMO baked chips. Enjoy with a side of no sugar added salsa. Pair with healthy protein, like a dollop of yogurt or hummus.
- Whole grain cereal, like steel cut oatmeal, topped with fresh berries or sliced fresh apple, and a dash of cinnamon
- Yogurt or Greek yogurt (unsweetened) with fresh fruit, like berries, and toasted sliced almonds

Chapter 26
Healthier Desserts and Treats

How to curb sweet cravings and replace sugary
desserts with satisfying, low glycemic treats.

Here are a few strategies to minimize the impact of desserts served on special occasions. You will also find ideas to help curb sweet cravings, as well as a few easy, delicious, low glycemic dessert recipes.

Curb sweet cravings with the scent of vanilla

To avoid a sweet craving after a meal, try sniffing pure vanilla extract. Researchers from St George's Hospital in London discovered that the scent of vanilla helps curb sweet cravings. In the study, people wearing wear a vanilla-scented patch had a significant decrease in their craving for sweets compared with those who did not wear the vanilla patch. Those with the vanilla scent also lost an average of four pounds in four weeks without dieting.

Researchers thought that the scent of vanilla may stimulate the release of the hunger-inhibiting hormone serotonin. The researchers said that biggest surprise in the study was that the vanilla scent was as effective in reducing cravings as some of the new weight-loss drugs, but without the side effects.

Before a sweet craving hits, reach for your favorite fresh fruit

If you know that a craving for sweets will hit you later in the day, *thirty minutes before a sweet craving hits,* reach for a piece of fresh fruit. Research shows that when people ate a piece of fruit thirty minutes before a craving hit, they were able to avoid the sweet craving. Reach for a piece of your favorite low-GI fruit, like a slice of fresh orange sprinkled with cinnamon or a few fresh berries.

Can exercise helps eliminate sweet cravings?

If you want to avoid cravings for sugary treats or dessert in the late day, engage in 15 minutes of exercise earlier in the day. Researchers in a PLOS ONE study discovered when people exercised for 15 minutes early in the day, they experienced a *significant decrease* in their cravings for sweet snacks later in the day.

How to plan for holidays and special events

Bring a healthier dessert

Sugary desserts are often served at holiday parties and special events. To avoid a carb or sugar overload, bring a healthier dessert to share, like a bowl of chilled mixed berries with freshly whipped low-sugar whipped cream. If the party or event is catered, ask if there is fresh fruit or another low-blood sugar impact option available.

Have "just a bite"

Once your blood sugar is in a healthy range, if you plan to have dessert on a special occasion, the American Diabetes Association recommends having "just a bite," or a small forkful from the front, middle, or back. You can have a small taste without overwhelming your body with a surge of sugar and fast carbohydrates. Ideally, pair with a healthy protein for fruit with fiber, like berries, nuts or almonds. Drinking water can also naturally help dilute the sugars.

How to keep sugars and fast carbs to a minimum

Keep foods high in added sugar and fast carbs to a minimum when starting a new eating plan. Here are a few low sugar dessert options:

Low Sugar, Low Carb Desserts

Apples with nut butter

Fresh apple slices topped with a dab of peanut butter or almond butter and roll in chopped nuts for a delicious low glycemic treat. Fresh apple slices are high in vitamin C and have beneficial apple pectin—an easy-to-digest fruit fiber that helps prevent a rise in blood sugar. Nuts contain beneficial healthy plant-based fats, but may also be high in extra calories. Use about 1/2 teaspoon of no-sugar-added peanut or almond butter on a slice of apple

Ingredients:
Fresh apple slices, like Honey Crisp apples
1/4 teaspoon unsweetened peanut butter or almond butter (per slice of fresh apple)
Crushed almonds or peanuts (to match the nut butter you choose)

Frozen fresh fruit

If you are looking for a refreshing frozen taste without added sugar, try having few pieces of frozen fresh fruit, like raspberries, strawberries, or fresh peach slices (without added sugar). Rinse frozen fruit under warm water for a minute or two until they start to thaw, and enjoy. It's like having a Popsicle with all of the goodness and flavor, but without added sugar.'

Ingredients:
Frozen fresh strawberries, fresh peach slices, raspberries (ideally organic)

Greek coconut yogurt with fruit and toasted almonds

Mix fresh coconut flakes into 1% or 2% unsweetened creamy Greek yogurt with fresh berries and toasted slivered almonds. Add unsweetened coconut flakes, and sprinkle of cinnamon for a little extra blood-sugar balancing power.

Ingredients:

1/2 cup creamy unsweetened Greek yogurt (2% or higher)
1/2 cup fresh berries, chopped
1 tablespoon unsalted toasted slivered almonds
1 teaspoon unsweetened coconut flakes
Cinnamon

Hearty trail mix

Trail mix without sugary ingredients is a crunchy, satisfying, low carb treat that is easy to make. Combine your favorite unsalted nuts and seeds, such as toasted pumpkin seeds, slivered almonds, and pecans in a small bowl. Add a few unsweetened coconut flakes and a sprinkle of cinnamon.

Ingredients:

1/2 cup unsalted mixed nuts, such as toasted almonds, walnut pieces, and pecans
1/2 cup unsalted mixed seeds, such as toasted pumpkin and sunflower seeds
1 tablespoon unsweetened coconut flakes (optional)

1 tablespoon low-sugar dried cranberries (optional)
1 tablespoon mini semisweet chocolate chips (optional)

Mocha ricotta dream dessert

To create this creamy low-sugar dessert, mix together: a half-cup of part-skim, low-calorie, ricotta cheese with 2 teaspoons of your favorite low glycemic chocolate or vanilla flavor protein powder (or 1 teaspoon of your favorite non-sugar sweetener), 1/2 teaspoon of unsweetened cocoa powder, 1/8 teaspoon of vanilla extract, and 1 teaspoon of brewed coffee. Top with fresh strawberries, a few dark chocolate chips, cinnamon, and toasted slivered almonds. The recommended serving size is about 1/2 cup.

Ingredients:

1/2 cup part-skim ricotta cheese
2 teaspoons low glycemic chocolate or vanilla protein powder (or 1 teaspoon of your favorite non-sugar sweetener)
1/2 teaspoon unsweetened cocoa powder (ideally non-Dutched)
1/8 teaspoon vanilla extract
1 teaspoon brewed coffee
1/2 cup fresh strawberries, chopped
Mini dark chocolate chips, 55% or higher

Pear and peach parfait

This fun parfait is a refreshing blood-sugar-friendly treat. Place a tablespoon of fresh chopped pears bottom of a small juice glass (but not high-sugar canned or packaged fruit), and then add a tablespoon or two of low-fat cottage or creamier full-fat cheese. Add a layer of freshly chopped peaches (but not high-sugar canned or packaged fruit), then another layer of cottage cheese. Top with toasted slivered almonds and a sprinkle of cinnamon. Other fresh low-sugar impact fruits you can use are fresh strawberries and blueberries.

Ingredients:

1/4 cup fresh pears, like Bosch pears, diced (but not overly ripe)
1/4 cup fresh peaches, diced (but not overly ripe)
1/2 cup creamy cottage cheese (2% or whole milk)
Crushed almonds or peanuts (to match the nut butter you choose)

Rich chocolate avocado pudding

Scoop out the flesh of two ripe avocados into a blender or food processor. Remove any dark spots in the flesh. Mix for 1 minute on high speed. Stop and scrape the avocado off of the sides back into the center of the blender. Blend again until avocado is smooth. Add unsweetened cocoa powder, cinnamon, coconut milk , sweetener, and vanilla extract. Blend again for a few second until mixed.

Taste and adjust sweetness by adding an additional teaspoon more of your favorite sugar-free monk fruit or monk fruit blended sweetener as needed. For a creamier, less thick pudding, add one teaspoon more of coconut milk or the milk or plant-based milk of your choice. Scoop into small ramekins or small glass jars and refrigerate for at least one hour before serving. The pudding can be stored in an airtight container in the fridge for up to 3 days. It tastes best when served fresh! Top with a sprinkle of toasted almonds or mini semisweet 55%+ chips before serving.

Ingredients:

2 avocados (flesh)

2 tablespoon unsweetened cocoa powder (ideally non-Dutched)

2-3 tablespoons monk fruit sweetener, or your favorite non-sugar sweetener (add to taste)

1 teaspoon low glycemic chocolate or vanilla protein powder (adds sweetness, optional)

1/2 cup coconut milk canned (full fat, not low fat)

1/2 teaspoon vanilla extract

1/8 teaspoon cinnamon

Dash of salt

Chapter 27
Superfood Drinks & Power Shake Recipes

*My favorite superfood drinks and
balancing protein shakes.*

Delicious power shakes with protein powder support healthy blood sugar. They also have balancing greens (you will hardly taste) and can even replace a meal!

Power greens

Green leafy vegetables are a powerhouse of vitamins, healing nutrients, and studies show, have a balancing effect on blood sugar. According to a study published in the *Journal of Diabetes Investigation*, they can also lower your risk of cancer, heart disease, and type 2 diabetes.

Kale

Kale is called a superfood for a reason. It's loaded with healthy nutrients. It's also one of the most energizing green leafy vegetables you can add to a shake. Among its many amazing health benefits, studies have found that kale may have a balancing influence on blood sugar and may help prevent diabetes.

The best way to add kale to a shake is to first blanch, and then freeze kale (without the stems) so it's ready to add when you make your shake. Blanching kale lessens its bitterness and preserves its healing nutrients, and frozen kale is easier to add to a shake. Kale can keep for up to 6 months in the freezer when properly stored in airtight freezer bags, according to experts from Eatingwell.com.

Tip! The easiest way to blanch kale is to remove the leaves from the stems, then separate or chop the leaves into bite-size pieces. Discard the stems. In a large pot, steam the kale for one or two minutes until it turns bright green, but not until its limp. Kale can also be blanched by boiling it directly in water for one to two minutes, but steaming it retains more healing nutrients. Drain well, cool, then freeze, separating the pieces in the container so it's easy to remove.

Organic barley grass powder

Barley grass powder is made from young organic barley grass. This nutrient-rich green superfood can help with digestion, and a recent National Institutes of Health study showed that barley grass may also improve insulin resistance.

Barley grass powder may have a balancing effect if you had more carbohydrates than you planned. It can also give you a boost if you feel a bit low energy. Try mixing a teaspoon of unsweetened or low-glycemic organic barley grass powder into a protein shake. It helps soothe digestion and supports healthy blood sugar.

Barley grass powder made from young barley grass has the most nutritional value, experts say. Avoid brands that have artificial sweeteners or added sugar.

Milk, almond milk

Adding milk, like 1% or 2% organic milk, or unsweetened almond milk adds protein and is a good base for a shake. You can also add another unsweetened plant-based milk, like oat milk.

Fresh fruit

Fresh or frozen low glycemic fruits, like strawberries, contain helpful antioxidants, fiber, and add refreshing flavor to your shake. The recommended serving size is typically about a ½ cup.

Whey protein powder

Protein powder is important to add to your shake. Whey is dairy-based and is a complete protein that contains all of the essential amino acids your body needs. It's naturally low in lactose, and studies suggest that whey protein may help support blood sugar. A European study found that when people had whey protein before a meal, they experienced fewer spikes in blood sugar after a meal.

Protein powder comes in delicious flavors, like strawberry, vanilla, and chocolate. Choose low glycemic, non-GMO protein powder with low glycemic sweeteners. You can find high-quality whey protein powders in health food stores and online.

If you prefer a non-dairy protein, pea protein is also a good choice.

Pea protein powder

Pea protein is a popular plant-based protein powder. While it's not a complete protein, studies suggest that pea protein may have a balancing effect on blood sugar levels. Look for pea protein powder, like Vanilla flavored pea protein that has low glycemic, naturally-derived sweeteners.

Cinnamon

Adding a generous dash of cinnamon can provide a little extra balancing power!

Power Shake Recipes

How to adjust ingredients:

Healthy greens, like kale and spinach, support healthy blood sugar.

Protein powder is also essential, as studies show that it can have a stabilizing effect. The studies show that people who had whey protein in the morning experienced fewer blood sugar spikes throughout the day.

A small scoop of your favorite *low glycemic* protein powder not only adds balancing protein, but helps sweeten your shake without causing a rapid rise in blood sugar.

Low glycemic vanilla or strawberry flavored protein powder compliments most shakes. Vanilla mixes with a variety of flavors, and strawberry is refreshing. Try a small package of different brands to find a flavor and brand you like that is sweetened with naturally-derived non-sugar sweeteners like stevia, erythritol, monk fruit, or a blend of no-sugar-impact natural sweeteners.

Protein powder is filling and can make your shake thick. You may not need an entire scoop to add flavor and protein. Start with a smaller portion, like a tablespoon or two. You can always add more if needed to sweeten your shake.

Also add up to ½ cup of your favorite fresh or frozen fruit, like strawberries. A ½ cup portion is recommended to lessen the impact of the natural sugars in the fruit. Enjoy!

Refreshing Strawberry Superfood Shake

Ingredients:

1 cup milk (low fat or 1%) or unsweetened almond milk

1/2 cup fresh or frozen strawberries

¼ cup chopped frozen kale (blanched)

1 teaspoon organic greens powder, such as barley grass powder (optional)

2 tablespoons of strawberry (or vanilla) flavored low glycemic protein powder

Generous dash of cinnamon

Directions:

1. Combine all ingredients in a blender.

2. Mix until smooth.

3. Add more liquid if the shake is too thick.

4. Add another teaspoon of low glycemic protein powder if needed for a sweeter taste.

Chocolate Lover's Superfood Shake

Ingredients:

1 cup milk (low fat or 1%) or unsweetened almond milk

1 teaspoon unsweetened cocoa powder

1/3 cup chopped kale (blanched)

1 teaspoon organic greens powder, such as barley grass
powder (optional)

2 tablespoons of chocolate-flavored low glycemic protein
powder

Generous dash of cinnamon

Directions:

1. Combine all ingredients in a blender.

2. Mix until smooth.

3. Add more liquid if the shake is too thick.

4. Add another teaspoon of low glycemic protein powder
if needed for a sweeter taste.

Strawberry Dream Protein Shake

Ingredients:

1 cup milk (low fat or 1%) or unsweetened almond milk

3/4 cup fresh or frozen strawberries. sliced

2 tablespoons of strawberry or vanilla flavored low
glycemic protein powder (or as needed to taste)

1 teaspoon wheat germ (adds whole grain fiber) (optional)

1/8 teaspoon vanilla extract

Generous dash of cinnamon

Directions:

1. Combine all ingredients in a blender.

2. Mix until smooth.

3. Add more liquid if the shake is too thick.

4. Add another teaspoon of low glycemic protein powder
if needed for a sweeter taste.

Refreshing Vanilla Peach Shake

Ingredients:

1 cup milk (low fat or 1%) or unsweetened almond milk
1/2 cup fresh or frozen unsweetened peaches
1 teaspoon wheat germ (adds whole grain fiber) (optional)
2 tablespoons of vanilla flavored, low glycemic protein
   powder (or as needed to taste)
1/4 teaspoon vanilla extract
Generous dash of cinnamon

Directions:

1. Combine all ingredients in a blender.
2. Mix until smooth.
3. Add more liquid if the shake is too thick.
4. Add another teaspoon of low glycemic protein powder if needed for a sweeter taste.

Vanilla Cream Superfood Shake

Ingredients:

1 cup milk (low fat or 1%) or unsweetened almond milk

1 tablespoon unsweetened yogurt (low fat or 2% for a
creamier taste)

1/4 cup chopped frozen kale (blanched)

1 teaspoon organic greens powder, such as barley grass
powder (optional)

2 tablespoons of vanilla flavored, low glycemic protein
powder (or as needed to taste)

1/4 teaspoon vanilla extract

Generous dash of cinnamon

Directions:

1. Combine all ingredients in a blender.

2. Mix until smooth.

3. Add more liquid if the shake is too thick.

4. Add another teaspoon of low glycemic protein powder
if needed for a sweeter taste.

Strawberry Peach Superfood Shake

Ingredients:

1 cup milk (low fat or 1%) or unsweetened almond milk

1 tablespoon unsweetened yogurt (2% for a creamier taste)

1/2 cup fresh or frozen strawberries. sliced

1/4 cup fresh or frozen sliced peaches

1 teaspoon wheat germ, adds sugar-balancing whole grain fiber and nutrients. (optional)

1/4 cup chopped frozen kale (blanched)

1 teaspoon organic greens powder, such as barley grass powder (optional)

2 tablespoons of strawberry or vanilla-flavored low glycemic protein powder (or as needed to taste)

Generous dash of cinnamon

Directions:

1. Combine all ingredients in a blender.

2. Mix until smooth.

3. Add more liquid if the shake is too thick.

4. Add another teaspoon of low glycemic protein powder if needed for a sweeter taste.

Coconut Strawberry Superfood Shake

Ingredients:

1 cup milk (low fat or 1%) or unsweetened almond milk

1 tablespoon unsweetened fresh coconut shavings

1/2 cup fresh or frozen strawberries

1/4 cup chopped frozen kale (blanched)

1 teaspoon organic greens powder, such as barley grass
powder (optional)

2 tablespoons of strawberry or vanilla-flavored, low
glycemic protein powder

Generous dash of cinnamon

Directions:

1. Combine all ingredients in a blender.

2. Mix until smooth.

3. Add more liquid if the shake is too thick.

4. Add another teaspoon of low glycemic protein powder
if needed for a sweeter taste.

Raspberry Cream Superfood Shake

Ingredients:
1 cup milk (low fat or 1%) or unsweetened almond milk
1 tablespoon unsweetened yogurt (low fat or 2% for a
    creamier taste)
1/3 cup fresh or frozen raspberries
1/4 cup chopped frozen kale (blanched)
1 teaspoon organic greens powder, such as barley grass
    powder (optional)
2 tablespoons of vanilla flavored low glycemic protein
    powder (to add protein and sweeten the shake)
Generous dash of cinnamon

Directions:
1. Combine all ingredients in a blender.
2. Mix until smooth.
3. Add more liquid if the shake is too thick.
4. Add another teaspoon of low glycemic protein powder
if needed for a sweeter taste.

Chapter 28
Your Body's Ability to Heal

The body has a tremendous ability to heal.

Knowledge is power

Your body is always working to stay healthy and keep everything running smoothly. When you lessen the carbohydrate and sugar load your body has to manage, maintain a healthy body weight, and eat a diet high in power healing foods and healing nutrients, you can strengthen your body systems and help them function better. A lifestyle that supports healthy blood sugar can refresh your health—and your blood sugar.

Knowledge is power. You will quickly discover what foods and food combinations work best for you, and those you may want to avoid entirely. And you can make any needed adjustments along the way.

Living a vibrant, healthy life

Every day is a new day to live a healthier, more vibrant life. You will be amazed at how much better you feel!

Chapter 29
To Your Good Health,
Author Note

Author note: To your good health!

I hope you found a natural path to refresh your health and blood sugar in these pages with delicious healing foods.

Inspiring Quotes

"Success is the sum of small efforts—repeated day in and day out."—Robert Collier

"You can't go back and change the beginning, but you can start where you are and change the ending."—James R. Sherman

About the Author

Find out more about the author and discover other media projects you may find interesting here:
www.paulaconstance.com.
Social Media @_paulaconstance.

If you found the information in this book helpful, please consider sharing a review.

Appendix A
12 Superfoods and
My Shopping List

12 Superfoods for healthy blood sugar

- **Almonds**: Almonds are low in carbs and high in protein
- **Apples:** Apples are high in natural pectin fiber, vitamin C, and important enzymes
- **Avocados:** Avocados are high in healthy vegetable fats, and are rich nutrients, with no cholesterol
- **Beans, Lentils:** Lentils and bean are high in fiber and help balance blood sugar
- **Berries:** Berries are low glycemic fruits with natural healthy fiber and beneficial antioxidants
- **Lemons, limes, grapefruit, oranges:** Citrus fruits are high in vitamin C and natural pulp and soluble fiber
- **Extra-Virgin Olive Oil:** Olive oil is high in healthy unsaturated vegetable fat and oemga-3s
- **Fish, Wild Salmon:** Salmon is high in omega-3 and healthy protein
- **Greek Yogurt:** Greek yogurt is a healthy protein
- **Kale and Spinach:** Kale and spinach are high in potent antioxidants and contain nutrients that stabilize blood sugar

- **Oats, Oat Bran:** Steel-cut oatmeal has oat bran and balancing natural fiber.
- **Pumpkin Seeds** Pumpkin seeds are naturally high in healthy fats that help balance blood sugar, have balancing fiber, and are a great choice.

My Shopping List

Here are a few of my favorite foods in every food category that can be part of a blood-sugar balancing lifestyle. Have fun and be creative!

Dairy and protein
- ✓ Cottage cheese, low fat or 2%
- ✓ Eggs
- ✓ Feta cheese (ideally, imported Greek feta)
- ✓ Low-fat cheese, such as part-skim mozzarella or low-fat Swiss cheese (avoid highly processed cheeses, like sliced American cheese)
- ✓ Milk, low fat, 1%, or 2% or almond milk
- ✓ Yogurt (like Greek yogurt, unsweetened, low-fat, or 2%)

Fruits
- ✓ Apples
- ✓ Avocados
- ✓ Blueberries
- ✓ Cherries
- ✓ Grapefruit
- ✓ Kiwis
- ✓ Lemons
- ✓ Limes
- ✓ Oranges
- ✓ Pears

My Shopping List

Here are a few of my favorite foods in every food category that can be part of a blood-sugar balancing lifestyle. Have fun and be creative!

Dairy and protein
- ✓ Cottage cheese, low fat or 2%
- ✓ Eggs
- ✓ Feta cheese (ideally, imported Greek feta)
- ✓ Low-fat cheese, such as part-skim mozzarella or low-fat Swiss cheese (avoid highly processed cheeses, like sliced American cheese)
- ✓ Milk, low fat, 1%, or 2% or almond milk
- ✓ Yogurt (like Greek yogurt, unsweetened, low-fat, or 2%)

Fruits
- ✓ Apples
- ✓ Avocados
- ✓ Blueberries
- ✓ Cherries
- ✓ Grapefruit
- ✓ Kiwis
- ✓ Lemons
- ✓ Limes
- ✓ Oranges
- ✓ Pears

✓ Raspberries
✓ Strawberries

Occasionally

✓ Banana (not overly ripe, a few slices). Bananas are a moderate impact fruit.

Veggies

✓ Artichokes
✓ Asparagus
✓ Avocado
✓ Beans, chickpeas, and lentils*
✓ Beets*
✓ Broccoli
✓ Brussels sprouts
✓ Butternut squash*
✓ Cabbage
✓ Cauliflower
✓ Carrot sticks
✓ Celery
✓ Corn on the cob*
✓ Cucumber
✓ Eggplant
✓ Kale
✓ Leafy greens
✓ Mushrooms
✓ Onions, scallions, leeks
✓ Peas, sugar snap peas*

- ✓ Peppers, red, green, yellow
- ✓ Radishes
- ✓ Spinach
- ✓ Sweet potatoes*
- ✓ Tomatoes
- ✓ Tomato sauce, tomato paste (no sugar added)
- ✓ Zucchini

***Note:** Beans, beets, butternut squash, corn, peas, and sweet potatoes may be higher in natural starches and carbs than other vegetables, but also contain healthy fiber that lessens the glycemic impact.

Lean Meat, Fish, and Seafood

- ✓ Chicken—ideally free-range, hormone and antibiotic-free)
- ✓ Fish, seafood—ideally wild-caught, up to 2x per week. (Limit tuna, swordfish, and other types of fish that may be high in mercury).
- ✓ Salmon—ideally wild-caught
- ✓ Sardines
- ✓ Tuna fish—ideally line-caught, dolphin-safe, and low in mercury
- ✓ Turkey—ideally antibiotic, hormone-free

Condiments, Pickles

- ✓ Balsamic vinegar, apple cider vinegar
- ✓ Cinnamon

- ✓ Ketchup—low-sugar brands, never with corn syrup
- ✓ Mayonnaise—Look for mayonnaise made with healthy oils, and avoid mayo with corn syrup.
- ✓ Mustard—without added sugar
- ✓ Pickles—with low or no added sugar. Avoid brands with corn syrup.
- ✓ Salsa—Many brands have no sugar or are very low in sugar (per serving). Salsa is made with delicious low-carb vegetables, such as tomatoes, peppers, and onions.
- ✓ Spices and herbs like oregano, basil, parsley, thyme, pepper, etc. Oregano and other spices have no sugar, add flavor, and often have tremendous health benefits.

Packaged, Jarred, and Prepared Foods
- ✓ Hummus—without added sugar
- ✓ Salsa—without added sugar
- ✓ Plant-based hamburger
- ✓ Soups—such as lentil, chicken, and vegetable soup, with low or no added sugar.
- ✓ Tomato sauce and tomato paste—without added sugar
- ✓ Veggie or plant-based burgers—look for brands low in sugar and carbs

Grains, Vegetable Pasta, Whole Grain Rice (not more than 1/2 cup cooked)
- ✓ Lentil pasta
- ✓ Quinoa

✓ Vegetable pasta, like zucchini pasta
✓ Whole grain rice (not more than a cup, cooked)

Cereal, Bread, and Crackers *(have a reasonable portion)*
✓ Almond flour crackers
✓ Bread—whole grain
✓ Cauliflower crackers
✓ Oatmeal
✓ Tortilla chips—whole grain, baked
✓ Shredded wheat cereal —without added sugar
✓ Whole grain cereal
✓ Wheat germ—ideally, toasted wheat germ*

*__Note:__ Wheat germ is made from the whole grain "germ" of the wheat (the germ is part of wheat that is often removed from refined wheat products, along with the husk, experts say). The germ is a nutritious whole grain food. Toasted wheat germ is often the cereal aisle but may sometimes be hard to find. You may have to ask where to find this nutritious, nutty-tasting, toasted cereal grain.

Frozen Foods
✓ Frozen low-carb veggie pizza with a thin whole grain or cauliflower crust (low in sugar and low-carb). Look for brands with a low sugar impact.
✓ Frozen sweet potato fries—no sugar added
✓ Frozen vegetables—such as broccoli, cauliflower, and mixed vegetables, without added sugar

Cooking Oil, Nuts, Seeds, and Popcorn
- ✓ Almonds, pecans, walnuts, all nuts
- ✓ Avocado oil
- ✓ Cashew butter, and other nut kinds of nut butter
- ✓ Coconut oil—not highly processed
- ✓ Flax seeds, pumpkin seeds, sunflower seeds, chia seeds, and sesame seeds
- ✓ Olive oil—ideally, extra virgin, first cold pressed
- ✓ Popcorn—ideally, air-popped. If you buy microwave popcorn, avoid artificial flavorings and unhealthy fats.
- ✓ Safflower oil—not highly processed

Ingredients and Spices
- ✓ Dark chocolate chips
- ✓ Natural vanilla extract
- ✓ Spices and herbs—Use creatively to flavor foods.

Appendix B
Lifestyle Checklist

Lifestyle checklist

1. Start every day ready to make it a healthy living day. Choose wholesome, healing foods and superfoods that support healthy blood sugar. Plan meals and snacks to support your wellness goals, and you are on your way!

2. Remember your "why." When you get up in the morning, remember why you want to make a change for the better. A new habit can become effortless in as few as 18 days, or 66 days on average, experts say. That's encouraging! And empowering. Choose a proven lifestyle plan that you are excited about and stay with it. Be honest with yourself. When something isn't working for you, decide how you can change it.

3 Stay with it. Give your healthy lifestyle plan 4 weeks and you should start to feel better. If you find yourself getting off track, start again. Also, find a like-minded health coach or wellness app to help provide a little extra motivation.

4 Try to maintain a healthy body weight. Even losing a few extra pounds can help improve your health, and blood sugar.

5. Start your morning with a nutritious breakfast. Eating a balanced breakfast in the morning can help prevent blood sugar spikes later in the day, researchers say.

6. Become mindfully aware of the foods you eat. Pay attention to how you feel about the foods you eat and how you feel after you eat. Are you satisfied with just the right portion? Do you feel more energized?

7. Pair carbohydrates with healthy protein. Protein helps slow the absorption of sugar.

8. Get enough sleep. When your body gets the rest it needs, it has a positive impact on your metabolism and blood sugar. If you didn't get enough sleep the night before, taking a short nap can help your body recharge.

9. Drink enough water. Staying hydrated helps all of your body systems function better.

10. Stay active! Only 30 minutes of healthy activity every day, like taking a brisk walk, or stretching every twenty minutes, has a positive impact on your health and blood sugar. Let's go!

References

"1 in 3 Adults Don't Get Enough Sleep." Centers for Disease Control and Prevention. Accessed February 6, 2019. https://www.cdc.gov/media/releases/2016/p0215-enough-sleep.html.

"7 Amazing Benefits of Safflower Oil." Organic Facts.net. Updated March 8, 2019. https://www.organicfacts.net/health-benefits/oils/safflower-oil.html.

"9 Things That Can Undermine Your Vitamin D Level." *Healthbeat* (blog). Health Publishing, Medical School. Accessed January 4, 2019. https://www.health.. edu/healthbeat/9-things-that-can-undermine-your-vitamin-d-level.

Adams, Case. "Pectin Slows Enzyme Activity and Absorption, Balancing Blood Sugar." Real Natural.org. Updated May 28, 2018. https://www.realnatural.org/pectin-slows-down-enzyme-activity-absorption-and-blood-sugar/.

Afkhami-Ardekani M, Shojaoddiny-Ardekani A. Effect of vitamin C on blood glucose, serum lipids & serum insulin in type 2 diabetes patients. Indian J Med Res. 2007 Nov;126(5):471-4. PMID: 18160753.

Ahmed AT, Karter AJ, Warton EM, Doan JU, Weisner CM. The relationship between alcohol consumption and glycemic control among patients with diabetes: the Kaiser Permanente Northern California Diabetes

Registry. J Gen Intern Med. 2008 Mar;23(3):275-82. doi: 10.1007/s11606-007-0502-z. Epub 2008 Jan 8. PMID: 18183468; PMCID: PMC2359478. https:// pubmed.ncbi.nlm.nih.gov/18183468/.

Ajala, Olubukola, Patrick English, and Jonathan Pinkney. "Systematic Review and Meta-Analysis of Different Dietary Approaches to the Management of Type 2 Diabetes." The American Journal of Clinical Nutrition. 97, no. 3 (March 2013): 505-516. https://academic.oup. com/ajcn/article/97/3/505/4571510#110493860.

"Alcohol." American Diabetes Association publication. Last Reviewed: September 30, 2013. Last Edited: June 6, 2014. https://myhealthonsite.com/wp-content/ uploads/2016/11/Alcohol-ADA.pdf. Reprinted with permission The American Diabetes Association. Copyright 2020 by the American Diabetes Association.

"Alcohol and Diabetes, Know the Risks." UCSF, Diabetes Center at the University of Southern California. Accessed December 11, 2020. https://diabetes.ucsf. edu/sites/diabetes.ucsf.edu/files/PEDS%20Alcohol%20 and%20Diabetes.pdf.

Alkaabi, J. M., Al-Dabbagh, B., Ahmad, S., Saadi, H. F., Gariballa, S., & Ghazali, M. A. (2011). Glycemic indices of five varieties of dates in healthy and diabetic subjects. Nutrition journal, 10, 59. https://doi. org/10.1186/1475-2891-10-59. https://www.ncbi.nlm. nih.gov/pmc/articles/PMC3112406/.

"All About the Grains Group." USDA United States Department of Agriculture. Choose My Plate. Accessed December 1, 2020. https://www.choosemyplate.gov/eathealthy/grains.

Almekinder, Elisabeth. "Can I Drink Milk If I Have Diabetes." The Diabetes Council.com Accessed February 24, 2020. https://www.thediabetescouncil.com/can-i-drink-milk-if-i-have-diabetes/.

Ambardekar, Nayana. "Diabetes and Alcohol." WedMD.com. Medically Reviewed May 11, 2019. https://www.webmd.com/diabetes/guide/drinking-alcohol#:~:text=While%20moderate%20amounts%20of%20alcohol,and%20may%20raise%20blood%20sugar.

Antoni, Rona, Tracey M. Robertson, M. Denise Robertson and Jonathan D. Johnston. Journal of Nutritional Science (2018), vol. 7, e22, page 1 of 6. "BRIEF REPORT: A pilot feasibility study exploring the effects of a moderate time-restricted feeding intervention on energy intake, adiposity and metabolic physiology in free-living human subjects." Accessed May 10, 2021. https://www.cambridge.org/core/services/aop-cambridge-core/content/view/S2048679018000137.

Apovian, Caroline, Susan McQuillan."Diabetic Diet: The Best Way to Eat for Type 2 Diabetes." EndocrineWeb.com. Accessed November 17, 2020. endocrineweb.com/conditions/diabetes/diabetes-diet-best-way-eat-type-2-diabetes.

"Are You on the Road to a Diabetes Diagnosis?" Health Publishing, Medical School, *Heart Letter*. February 2017. Updated December 12, 2019. https://www.health..edu/heart-health/are-you-on-the-road-to-a-diabetes-diagnosis.

Arnarson, Atli. "10 Evidence-Based Health Benefits of Whey Protein." Healthline.com. Accessed May 6, 2019. https://www.healthline.com/nutrition/10-health-benefits-of-whey-protein.

Anne, Melodie. "Glycemic Index of Honey vs. Sugar." Livestrong.com. Accessed March 10, 2019. https://www.livestrong.com/article/270875-honey-vs-sugar-glycemic-index/.

"Are Peas Good for Diabetes?" The Diabetes Council.com. Updated October 5, 2018. https://www.thediabetescouncil.com/are-peas-good-for-diabetes/.

Armour, Elizabeth. "How Many Almonds in a Serving?" FoodNetwork.com. Accessed January 14, 2019. https://www.foodnetwork.com/healthyeats/healthy-tips/2013/04/how-many-almonds-in-a-serving.

Arnarson, Atli. "Seven Benefits of Almond Milk." Medical News Today.com. August 1, 2017. https://www.medicalnewstoday.com/articles/318612.php.

Asp, M. L., Collene, A. L., Norris, L. E., Cole, R. M., Stout, M. B., Tang, S. Y., Hsu, J. C., & Belury, M. A. (2011). Time-dependent effects of safflower oil to improve glycemia, inflammation and blood lipids in obese, post-menopausal women with type 2 diabetes: a randomized, double-masked, crossover study. Clinical nutrition (Edinburgh, Scotland), 30(4), 443–449. https://www.ncbi.nlm.nih.gov/pmc/articles/PMC3115398/.

"Avoid The Hidden Dangers of High Fructose Corn Syrups." The Cleveland Clinic, December 1, 2020. https://health.clevelandclinic.org/avoid-the-hidden-dangers-of-high-fructose-corn-syrup-video/#:~:text=High%20fructose%20corn%20syrup%20has,diabetes%20and%20high%20blood%20pressure.

"Barley Grass." Drugs.com. Last updated on Jan 6, 2019. https://www.drugs.com/npc/barley-grass.html.Batra, Sukhsatej. "What Are the Benefits of Cold-Pressed Olive Oil?" Live Strong.com. Accessed August 14, 2017. https://www.livestrong.com/article/126478 benefits-cold-pressed-olive-oil/.

Bauer, Brent A. "What is BPA, and What Are the Concerns About BPA?" The Mayo Clinic. Accessed January 3, 2019. https://www.mayoclinic.org/healthy-lifestyle/nutrition-and-healthy-eating/expert-answers/bpa/faq-20058331.

Bazzano LA, Li TY, Joshipura KJ, Hu FB. Intake of fruit, vegetables, and fruit juices and risk of diabetes in women. Diabetes Care. 2008;31(7):1311-1317. doi:10.2337/dc08-0080

"Bean Accounting: Are Soy-Based Foods Products as Safe and Healthy as Advertised?" Scientific American. com. Accessed December 19, 2018. https://www. scientificamerican.com/article/how-safe-is-soy/.

Berkheiser, Kaitlyn "Magnesium Dosage: How Much Should You Take per Day?" July 6, 2018. https://www. healthline.com/nutrition/magnesium-dosage.

Bernard, Neal (2015, January 22) "A Plant-Based Diet Causes Weight Loss, According to New Mega-Study: People who Go Vegetarian Lose Weight without Counting Calories." George Washington School of Medicine and Health Sciences. Accessed May 6, 2019. https://smhs.gwu.edu/news/plant-based-diet-causes-weight-loss-according-new-mega-study.

"Bisphenol A (BPA): Use in Food Contact Application." US Food and Drug Administration. Updated June 27, 2018. https://www.fda.gov/newsevents/ publichealthfocus/ucm064437.htm.

Biggers, Alana. Scott Frothingham. "Diabetes and Corn Consumption: Is It OK?" February 1, 2019. https:// www.healthline.com/health/diabetes-corn.

"Blood Pressure Drugs Can Boost Blood Sugar." Health Publishing, Medical School, Heart Letter. February 2007. https://www.health..edu/newsletter_article/ blood-pressure-drugs-can-boost-blood-sugar.

"Blood Sugar Testing, Why, When, and How." The Mayo Clinic. Accessed June 23, 2020. https://www.mayoclinic.org/diseases-conditions/diabetes/in-depth/blood-sugar/art-20046628.

"Blood Sugar and Exercise." The American Diabetes Association Diabetes.org. Accessed January 29, 2022. https://www.diabetes.org/healthy-living/fitness/getting-started-safely/blood-glucose-and-exercise#:~:text=Physical%20activity%20can%20lower%20your,see%20the%20benefits%20of%20activity..

"Blue Tortillas May Help Dieters and Diabetics." ScienceDaily. Accessed August 1, 2007. https://www.sciencedaily.com/releases/2007/07/070730092559.htm.

"Boost the Immune System." University of Maryland Medical System. Accessed October 12, 2020. https://www.umms.org/coronavirus/what-to-know/managing-medical-conditions/healthy-habits/boost-immune-system#:~:text=Vitamin%20D%20is%20one%20of,risk%20of%20colds%20and%20flu.

"Breakfast: Is It the Most Important Meal?" WebMD.com. Accessed January 19, 2019. https://www.webmd.com/food-recipes/breakfast-lose-weight#1.

Brusso, Jessica. "Do Grapes Raise Blood Sugar?" Healthy Eating (blog) SFGate.com. Updated December 6, 2018. https://healthyeating.sfgate.com/grapes-raise-blood-sugar-3477.html.

Bucklin, Stephanie. "The Best Ways to Enjoy Dark Chocolate When You Have Diabetes." Every Day Health.com. Updated October 17, 2017. https://www.everydayhealth.com/type-2-diabetes/diet/why-dark-chocolate-one-best-desserts-diabetics/.

"Bulgur." Bobsredmill.com. Accessed November 30, 2020. https://www.bobsredmill.com/blog/healthy-living/is-kamut-gluten-free/.

Burgess, Lana. "Can You Have Hypoglycemia Without Diabetes?" Medical News Today.com. August 10, 2018. https://www.medicalnewstoday.com/articles/322744.php.

Butler, Natalie. Jerisha Parker Gordon. "Can I Eat Watermellon if I Have Diabetes?" September 27, 2016. https://www.healthline.com/health/diabetes/watermelon-and-diabetes.

Butler, Natalie. Annette McDermott. "Why Everyone's Going Mad for Monk Fruit." February 3, 2017. https://www.healthline.com/health/food-nutrition/monk-fruit-health-benefits.

Byrne, Jennifer. "What Are the Dangers of GMO Soybeans?" Livestrong.com. Accessed May 6, 2019. https://www.livestrong.com/article/200114-what-are-the-dangers-of-gmo-soybeans/.

Cafasso, Jacquelyn. "Agave Nectar vs. Honey: Which Is Healthier?" Healthline.com. Updated October 4, 2016.

https://www.healthline.com/health/food-nutrition/
agave-nectar-vs-honey.

Caffrey, Mary. "American Diabetes Association
Issues Recommendations for Physical Activity,
Exercise." October 31, 2016. https://www.ajmc.com/
newsroom/american-diabetes-association-issues-
recommendations-for-physical-activity-exercise.

Callahan, Alice. "7 Common Medicines That May Make
It Harder to Control Your Blood Sugar." Everyday
Health.com. Updated March 6, 2018. https://www.
everydayhealth.com/type-2-diabetes/treatment/
medications-may-affect-blood-sugar-control-diabetes/.

Campbell, Amy. "Low Carb Myths and Facts."
DiabetesSelfManagement.com. Accessed February 11,
2019. https://www.diabetesselfmanagement.com/blog/
low carb-myths-and-facts/.

"Can I Eat Pasta If I Have Diabetes?" The Diabetes
Council.com. The Diabetes Council Team. Accessed on
03/08/20. https://www.thediabetescouncil.com/can-i-
eat-pasta-if-i-have-diabetes/.

"Cantaloupe." DefeatDiabetes.org. Accessed October 7,
2018. https://defeatdiabetes.org/resources/healthful-
eating/fruits/cantaloupe-musk-melon/.

"Carbohydrates and Blood Sugar." The Nutrition
Source (blog). T.H. Chan School of Public Health.
Accessed September 7, 2020. https://www.hsph..edu/

nutritionsource/carbohydrates/carbohydrates-and-blood-sugar/#:~:text=When%20people%20eat%20a%20food,sugar%20for%20energy%20or%20storage.

"Carbohydrates Counting and Diabetes." The National Institute of Diabetes and Digestive and Kidney Diseases (NIDDK). Accessed January 15, 2020. https://www.niddk.nih.gov/health-information/diabetes/overview/diet-eating-physical-activity/carbohydrate-counting.

"Carbohydrates: How Carbs Fit Into a Healthy Diet." The Mayo Clinic. Accessed November 27, 2020. https://www.mayoclinic.org/healthy-lifestyle/nutrition-and-healthy-eating/in-depth/carbohydrates/art-20045705.

Carey, Elea. "10 Low glycemic Fruits for Diabetics." Healthline.com. August 18, 2017. www.healthline.com/health/diabetes/low glycemic-fruits-for-diabetes.

"Carrots and Their Effect on Blood Sugar." WebMD." Accessed October 4, 2020. https://www.webmd.com/diabetes/carrots-effect-on-blood-sugar#:~:text=Raw%20carrots%20have%20a%20GI,Low%20glycemic%20index%3A%201%2D55/.

Castro, M. Regina. "Caffeine: Does it affect blood sugar?" Mayo Clinic. Accessed March 21, 2020. https://www.mayoclinic.org/diseases-conditions/type-2-diabetes/expert-answers/blood-sugar/faq-20057941.

Castro, M. Regina. "Is it True That Cinnamon Can Lower Blood Sugar in People Who Have Diabetes?" Mayo Clinic. Accessed May 6, 2019. https://www.mayoclinic.org/diseases-conditions/diabetes/expert-answers/diabetes/faq-20058472.

"Catching up on Sleep." The National Sleep Foundation. Sleep.org. Accessed September 25, 2019. https://www.sleep.org/articles/catching-up-on-sleep/.

Chaparro, Marina. "Pasta and Diabetes: 5 Healthy Ways to Eat Pasta." Updated August 29, 2018. OnTrackDiabetes.com https://www.ontrackdiabetes.com/live-well/eat-well/pasta-diabetes-5-healthy-ways-eat-pasta.

"Checking Your Blood Glucose." Diabetes.org. Updated October 9, 2018. http://www.diabetes.org/living-with-diabetes/treatment-and-care/blood-glucose-control/checking-your-blood-glucose.html.

Chenjuan Gu, Nga Brereton, Amy Schweitzer, Matthew Cotter, Daisy Duan, Elisabet Børsheim, Robert R Wolfe, Luu V Pham, Vsevolod Y Polotsky, Jonathan C Jun."Metabolic Effects of Late Dinner in Healthy Volunteers—A Randomized Crossover Clinical Trial." The Journal of Clinical Endocrinology & Metabolism, Volume 105, Issue 8, August 2020, Pages 2789–2802, https://doi.org/10.1210/clinem/dgaa354

Cherney, Kristeen. "All of the Health Benefits of Sweet Potatoes for People with Diabetes." Ecom. Updated November 10, 2017. https://www.everydayhealth.

com/type-2-diabetes/diet/top-health-benefits-sweet-potatoes-diabetics/.

"Choosing Oils for Cooking: A Host of Heart Healthy Options." *Heart Health*. March, 2019. "https://www.health..edu/heart-health/choosing-oils-for-cooking-a-host-of-heart-healthy-options."

Chudnovskiy R, Thompson A, Tharp K, Hellerstein M, Napoli JL, Stahl A. Consumption of clarified grapefruit juice ameliorates high-fat diet induced insulin resistance and weight gain in mice. PLOS One. 2014;9(10):e108408. Published 2014 Oct 8. doi:10.1371/journal.pone.0108408

Charles, Dan. "As Weeds Outsmart The Latest Weedkillers, Farmers Are Running Out Of Easy Options." NPR, Morning Edition. April 11, 201. https://www.npr.org/sections/thesalt/2019/04/11/710229186/as-weeds-outsmart-the-latest-weedkillers-farmers-are-running-out-of-options.

Chiles, Andy. " Reading Can Help Reduce Stress, According to University of Sussex Research."The Argus Newspaper. March 30, 2009. https://www.theargus.co.uk/news/4245076.reading-can-help-reduce-stress-according-to-university-of-sussex-research/.

Church, Kacy. Fetters, Aleisha Fetters. " How Exercise Helps Prevent and Manage Type 2 Diabetes."September 15, 2020. Everyday Health. https://www.everydayhealth.com/type-2-diabetes/how-exercise-helps-prevent-and-manage-type-2-diabetes/.

"Cinnamon and Cassia." The Food and Agriculture Organization. Accessed June 14, 2020. http://www. fao.org/3/x5326e/x5326e07.htm#2.%20cinnamon%20 and%20cassia.

"Cinnamon and Diabetes." Diabetes.co.uk. Accessed November 11, 2019. https://www.diabetes.co.uk/ natural-therapies/cinnamon.html

"Circadian Rhythms." National Institute of General Medical Sciences, National Institutes of Health. Accessed September 14, 2020. https://www.nigms.nih. gov/education/fact-sheets/Pages/circadian-rhythms. aspx.

Cohen, Holly. "Oat Milk: What to Know About This Dairy-Free Alt-Milk." USnews.com. Aug. 9, 2018. https:// health.usnews.com/wellness/food/articles/2018-08-09/ oat-milk-what-to-know-about-this-dairy-free-alt-milk.

Cohen, Suzy. "The Surprising Connection Between Stevia and Ragweed."SuzyCohen.com. Accessed August 6, 2020. https://suzycohen.com/articles/stevia_ragweed/.

Coleman, Erin. "How Much Protein Is There in 10 Almonds?" SFGate.com. Updated November 19, 2018. https://healthyeating.sfgate.com/much-protein-there-10-almonds-6036.html.

Collier, Robert. Quote used with permission. With special thanks to Robert Collier Publications LLC. http://www.RobertCollierpublications.com.

Coyle, Daisy. "Starchy vs Non-Starchy Vegetables: Food Lists and Nutrition Facts." Healthline.com. October 3, 2018. https://www.healthline.com/nutrition/starchy-vs-non-starchy-vegetables.

"Consuming Milk at Breakfast Lowers Blood Glucose Throughout the Day: Effects of Protein Composition and Concentration." Science Daily.com. Accessed December 2, 2018. www.sciencedaily.com/releases/2018/08/180820085243.htm.

"Consuming Whey Protein Before Meals Could Help Improve Blood Glucose Control in People with Diabetes." ScienceDaily. Accessed May 6, 2019. https://www.sciencedaily.com/releases/2014/07/140707212746.htm.

Corleone, Jill. "Can Diabetics Eat Plums?" SFGate.com. Updated November 27, 2018. https://healthyeating.sfgate.com/can-diabetics-eat-plums-10633.html.

Corleone, Jill. Karen, Gardner. "The Pros and Cons of Safflower Oil." Livestrong.com. July 5, 2019 . https://www.livestrong.com/article/546738-the-pros-cons-of-safflower-oil/.

Cotton, Meredith. "Sources of Glucose." Kaiser Permanente, *Health and Wellness*. January 3,

2019. https://wa-search.kaiserpermanente.org/vis/cgi-bin/query-meta?v:project=ghc-ext-PublicProject&query=sources%20of%20glucose.

"Cranberry Juice Chemicals Could Cut Risk of Heart Disease and Type 2 Diabetes. July 1, 2015. Diabetes.co.uk. http://www.diabetes.co.uk/news/2015/jul/cranberry-juice-chemicals-could-cut-risk-of-heart-disease-and-type-2-diabetes-91211084.html.

Crosby, Guy. "Ask The Expert: Concerns About Canola Oil." The Nutrition Source (blog). T.H. Chan School of Public Health. Updated December 2018. https://www.hsph..edu/nutritionsource/2015/04/13/ask-the-expert-concerns-about-canola-oil/.

"Cut Down on Added Sugars." Dietary Guidelines for Americans (2015-2020) Eighth Edition. Accessed December 19, 2019. https://health.gov/dietaryguidelines/2015/resources/DGA_Cut-Down-On-Added-Sugars.pdf

De Long, Nicole E, and Alison C Holloway. "Early-Life Chemical Exposures and Risk of Metabolic Syndrome." Diabetes, Metabolic Syndrome and Obesity: Targets and Therapy vol. 10 101-109. 21 Mar. 2017, doi:10.2147/DMSO.S95296.

De Lordes Lima M, Cruz T, Pousada JC, Rodrigues LE, Barbosa K, Canguçu V. "The Effect of Magnesium Supplementation in Increasing Doses on the Control of Type 2 Diabetes." Diabetes Care. 1998 May;21(5):682-6. PubMed PMID: 9589224.

Dean I, Jackson F, Greenough RJ. Chronic (1-year) oral toxicity study of erythritol in dogs. Regul Toxicol Pharmacol. 1996 Oct;24(2 Pt 2):S254-60. doi: 10.1006/rtph.1996.0106. PMID: 8933641.

"Diabetes and Carbs." Centers for Disease Control and Prevention. Accessed June 20, 2020. https://www.cdc.gov/diabetes/managing/eat-well/diabetes-and-carbohydrates.html#:~:text=Try%20to%20limit%20foods%20that,A%20small%20piece%20of%20fruit.

Diabetes." Mayo Clinic. Accessed May 6, 2019. https://www.mayoclinic.org/diseases-conditions/diabetes/diagnosis-treatment/drc-20371451.

"Diabetes and Carbs." The US Centers for Disease Control and Prevention. September 19, 2019. https://www.cdc.gov/diabetes/managing/eat-well/diabetes-and-carbohydrates.html.

"Diabetes and Milk." Diabetes NSW & Act. Tuesday, 30 July 2019. https://diabetesnsw.com.au/about-us/blog/what-type-of-milk-is-right-for-me/#:~:text=Made%20from%20grains%2C%20oat%20milk,choice%20for%20people%20with%20diabetes.

"Diabetes and Mindfulness." Diabetes.co.uk. Accessed October 7, 2018. https://www.diabetes.co.uk/emotions/diabetes-and-mindfulness.html.

"Diabetes and Your Heart." CDC, Centers for Disease Control and Prevention. Accessed September

14, 2020. https://www.cdc.gov/diabetes/library/
features/diabetes-and-heart.html#:~:text=Over%20
time%2C%20high%20blood%20sugar,and%20can%20
damage%20artery%20walls.

Diabetes Prevention Program Research Group. "Reduction
in the Incidence of Type 2 Diabetes with Lifestyle
Intervention or Metformin." The New England Journal
of Medicine 2002, 346: 393-403. https://www.nejm.org/
doi/full/10.1056/NEJMoa012512.

"Diabetic Hypoglycemia." Mayo Clinic. Accessed February
7, 2019. https://www.mayoclinic.org/diseases-
conditions/diabetic-hypoglycemia/symptoms-causes/
syc-20371525.

"Diabetes Remission." Diabetes Remission in People with
Type 2 Diabetes Means that Your Blood Sugar Levels
are Healthy Without Needing to Take any Diabetes
Medication. Diabetes.org. Accessed December 8,
2020. https://www.diabetes.org.uk/guide-to-diabetes/
managing-your-diabetes/treating-your-diabetes/type2-
diabetes-remission.

"Diabetes Symptoms: When Diabetes Symptoms
Are a Concern." Accessed December 7, 2020.
https://www.mayoclinic.org/diseases-conditions/
diabetes/in-depth/diabetes-symptoms art-
20044248#:~:text=Excessive%20thirst%20and%20
increased%20urination%20are%20common%20
diabetes%20signs%20and,and%20absorb%20the%20
excess%20glucose.

"Diagnosing Diabetes and Learning About Prediabetes." The American Diabetes Association. Updated November 21, 2016. http://www.diabetes.org/diabetes-basics/diagnosis/. Reprinted with permission The American Diabetes Association. Copyright 2020 by the American Diabetes Association.

DiCorleto, Paul. "Why You Should Pay Attention to Chronic Inflammation: The Connection Between Inflammation and Disease." Cleveland Clinic, Health Essentials, *Cancer Care*. October 14, 2014. https://health.clevelandclinic.org/why-you-should-pay-attention-to-chronic-inflammation/.

"Dietary Fiber Essential for a Healthy Diet." Mayo Clinic. Accessed January 17, 2020. https://www.mayoclinic.org/healthy-lifestyle/nutrition-and-healthy-eating/in-depth/fiber/art-20043983.

"Dietary Guidelines 2015-2020." Executive Summary, *Key Recommendations*. Accessed December 5, 2020. https://health.gov/our-work/food-nutrition/2015-2020-dietary-guidelines/guidelines/executive-summary/.

"Dietary Reference Intakes for Calcium and Vitamin D." Institute of Medicine of the National Academies. Revised March 2011. http://www.nationalacademies.org/hmd/~/media/Files/Report%20Files/2010/Dietary-Reference-Intakes-for-Calcium-and-Vitamin-D/Vitamin%20D%20and%20Calcium%202010%20Report%20Brief.pdf.

Dita Moravek, Alison M Duncan, Laura B VanderSluis, Sarah J Turkstra, Erica J Rogers, Jessica M Wilson, Aileen Hawke, D Dan Ramdath, Carbohydrate Replacement of Rice or Potato with Lentils Reduces the Postprandial Glycemic Response in Healthy Adults in an Acute, Randomized, Crossover Trial, The Journal of Nutrition, Volume 148, Issue 4, April 2018, Pages 535–541, https://doi.org/10.1093/jn/nxy018

Doheny, Kathleen. "Skipping Breakfast: Bad Idea for People With Type 2 Diabetes." EndocrineWeb. com. Updated December 5, 2017. https://www. endocrineweb.com/news/diabetes/17894-skipping-breakfast-bad-idea-people-type-2-diabetes.

Dubey, P., Kumar, Y., Singh, R., Jha, K., & Kumar, R. (2019). Effect of music of specific frequency upon the sleep architecture and electroencephalographic pattern of individuals with delayed sleep latency: A daytime nap study. Journal of family medicine and primary care, 8(12), 3915–3919. https://doi.org/10.4103/jfmpc. jfmpc_575_19.

Dutton, Eileen. "Clean Eating, What Does it Mean?" The Mayo Clinic, *Speaking of Health* blog. September 12, 2019. https://www.mayoclinichealthsystem.org/ hometown-health/speaking-of-health/clean-eating-what-does-that-mean.

Du, H., Li, L., Bennett, D., Guo, Y., Turnbull, I., Yang, L., Bragg, F., Bian, Z., Chen, Y., Chen, J., Millwood, I. Y., Sansome, S., Ma, L., Huang, Y., Zhang, N., Zheng, X., Sun, Q., Key, T. J., Collins, R., Peto, R., …

China Kadoorie Biobank study (2017). Fresh fruit consumption in relation to incident diabetes and diabetic vascular complications: A 7-y prospective study of 0.5 million Chinese adults. PLoS medicine, 14(4), e1002279. https://doi.org/10.1371/journal.pmed.1002279.

"Eat Any Sugar Alcohol Lately?" Yale New Haven Hospital, Yale New Haven Nutrition, Health. Accessed June 9, 2020. https://www.ynhh.org/services/nutrition/sugar-alcohol.aspx#:~:text=Sugar%20alcohols%2C%20also%20know%20as,such%20as%20fruits%20and%20berries.

Edwards, Helen. "Making Rice Nice for Diabetes." Your Diabetes Hub (blog), January 12, 2015. https://www.yourdiabeteshub.com/making-rice-nice-diabetes/.

Edwards, Michael. "Healthy Sugar Alternatives & More." Organic Lifestyle Magazine, June 12, 2007. Updated July 23, 2017. www.organiclifestylemagazine.com/healthy-sugar-alternatives-more.

Ellis TP, Wright AG, Clifton PM, Ilag LL. Postprandial insulin and glucose levels are reduced in healthy subjects when a standardised breakfast meal is supplemented with a filtered sugarcane molasses concentrate. Eur J Nutr. 2016 Dec;55(8):2365-2376. doi: 10.1007/s00394-015-1043-6. Epub 2015 Sep 26. PMID: 26410392. Emanuele, N V et al. "Consequences of alcohol use in diabetics." Alcohol health and research world vol. 22,3 (1998): 211-9. https://pubmed.ncbi.nlm.nih.gov/26410392/.

Endocrine Society. "Napping reverses health effects of poor sleep, study finds." ScienceDaily. www.sciencedaily. com/releases/2015/02/150210141734.htm (accessed October 30, 2020).

Esposito, Katherine, Maria Ida Maiorino, Michela Petrizzo, Giuseppe Bellastella, and Dario Giugliano. "The Effects of a Mediterranean Diet on the Need for Diabetes Drugs and Remission of Newly Diagnosed Type 2 Diabetes: Follow-up of a Randomized Trial." Diabetes Care 37, no. 7 (July 2014): 1824-1830. http://care. diabetesjournals.org/content/37/7/1824.

"Extra Weight, Extra Risk." The American Diabetes Association. Accessed January 8, 2020. https://www. diabetes.org/diabetes-risk/prevention/overweight.

Evangelou, Evangelos, Georgios Ntritsos, Maria Chondrogiorgi, Fotini K. Kavvoura, Antonio F. Hernández, Evangelia E. Ntzani, and Ioanna Tzoulaki. "Exposure to Pesticides and Diabetes: A Systematic Review and Meta-Analysis." Environment International 91 (May 2016): 60-68. https://www.sciencedirect.com/ science/article/pii/S0160412016300496?via%3Dihub.

Falck, Suzanne, James Roland. "What You Should Know About Diabetes and Beans." Healthline.com. October 30, 2017. https://www.healthline.com/health/diabetes/ beans#1.

Fetters, Aleisha K. "What Are Greens Powders–And Do You Need Them?" US News and World Report, November 17, 2017. https://health.usnews.com/

wellness/food/articles/2017-11-17/what-are-greens-powders-and-do-you-need-them.

"First Cold Pressed –What Does It Mean?" TexasOliveRanch.com. August 17, 2017. "https://texasoliveranch.com/olive-oil-education/first-cold-pressed-what-does-it-mean/.

Fletcher, Jenna. "Can People with Diabetes Eat Popcorn?" MedicalNewsToday.com. Updated March 26, 2019. https://www.medicalnewstoday.com/articles/317330.php.

"Food Data Central." United States Department of Agriculture, USDA. Accessed January 1, 2021. https://fdc.nal.usda.gov/.

"Food Order Has Significant Impact on Glucose and Insulin Levels." Well Cornell Medicine. Accessed August 28, 2019. https://news.weill.cornell.edu/news/2015/06/food-order-has-significant-impact-on-glucose-and-insulin-levels-louis-aronne

"Foods That Fight Inflammation." Medical School, Health Publishing, *Women's Health Watch*. Updated August 29, 2020. https://www.health.harvard.edu/staying-healthy/foods-that-fight-inflammation.

Franz MJ. Protein: metabolism and effect on blood glucose levels. Diabetes Educ. 1997 Nov-Dec;23(6):643-6, 648, 650-1. doi: 10.1177/014572179702300603. PMID: 9416027.

Fumiaki Imamura, Renata Micha,Jason H. Y. Wu, Marcia C. de Oliveira Otto, Fadar O. Otite,Ajibola I. Abioye, Dariush Mozaffarian. Effects of Saturated Fat, Polyunsaturated Fat, Monounsaturated Fat, and Carbohydrate on Glucose-Insulin Homeostasis: A Systematic Review and Meta-analysis of Randomized Controlled Feeding Trials. Published: July 19, 2016. https://doi.org/10.1371/journal.pmed.1002087.

Furmli S, Elmasry R, Ramos M, et al Therapeutic use of intermittent fasting for people with type 2 diabetes as an alternative to insulin. Case Reports 2018;2018:bcr-2017-221854.

Franz, MJ. "Protein: Metabolism and Effect on Blood Glucose Levels." The Diabetes Educator. 1997 Nov-Dec; 23(6):643-6, 648, 650-1. https://www.ncbi.nlm.nih.gov/pubmed/9416027.

Gardner, B., Lally, P., & Wardle, J. (2012). Making health habitual: the psychology of 'habit-formation' and general practice. The British journal of general practice : the journal of the Royal College of General Practitioners, 62(605), 664–666. https://doi.org/10.3399/bjgp12X659466. https://www.ncbi.nlm.nih.gov/pmc/articles/PMC3505409/.

Gardner, Sarah and Albee, Dave, "Study focuses on strategies for achieving goals, resolutions" (2015). Press Releases. 266.https://scholar.dominican.edu/news-releases/266

Gasnier C1, Dumont C, Benachour N, Clair E, Chagnon MC, Séralini GE. "Glyphosate-based Herbicides are Toxic and Endocrine Disruptors in Human Cell Lines." Toxicology. 2009 Aug 21;262(3):184-91. doi: 10.1016/j.tox.2009.06.006. Epub 2009 Jun 17.

Gebel, Erica. "The Role of Sleep in Type 2 Diabetes." Diabetes Forecast. May 2011. http://www.diabetesforecast.org/2011/may/the-role-of-sleep-in-type-2-diabetes.html.

Geddes, Geoff. "GMO vs.Non-GMO Soybeans: A Growing Debate." North Star Genetics, November 15, 2016. https://www.northstargenetics.com/ca/2016/11/15/gmo-vs-non-gmo-soybeans-a-growing-debate/.

Geller, Samara and Sonya Lunder. "BPA in Canned Foods." Environmental Working Group, June 3, 2015. https://www.ewg.org/research/bpa-canned-food.

Gentile, Julie M. "Portion Control When You Have Type 2 Diabetes: Watching How Much You Eat." Ontrack Diabetes.com. Updated December 10, 2012. https://www.ontrackdiabetes.com/eating-well/portion-control-when-you-have-type-2-diabetes.

Georgoulis, Michael, Meropi D. Kontogianni, and Nikos Yiannakouris. "Mediterranean Diet and Diabetes: Prevent and Treatment." Special Issue, Nutrients: Mediterranean Diet Pattern and Public Health 6, no. 4 (2014): 1406-1423. https://www.mdpi.com/2072-6643/6/4/1406.

"Gi Database of Foods," The Glycemic Index Foundation. Accessed December 24, 2020. https://www.gisymbol. com/gi-database-of-foods/.

Gifford, Maria. "Type 2 Diabetes: Why Sleep Quality Matters." EverydayHealth.com. Accessed September 29, 2019. https://www.everydayhealth.com/hs/ type-2-diabetes-guide-healthy-habits/sleep-quality- matters/#targetText=The%20AACE%20says%20 that%20cardiometabolic,hours%20of%20sleep%20 each%20night.

Gillezeau, C., van Gerwen, M., Shaffer, R. M., Rana, I., Zhang, L., Sheppard, L., & Taioli, E. (2019). The evidence of human exposure to glyphosate: a review. Environmental health: a global access science source, 18(1), 2. https://doi.org/10.1186/s12940-018-0435- 5. https://www.ncbi.nlm.nih.gov/pmc/articles/ PMC6322310/.

"Glycemic Index." Self Nutrition Data. Nutritiondata.self. com. Accessed May 6, 2019. https://nutritiondata.self. com/topics/glycemic-index.

"Glycemic Index for 60+ Foods." Health Publishing, Medical School. Updated March 14, 2018. https://www. health..edu/diseases-and-conditions/glycemic-index- and-glycemic-load-for-100-foods.

"Gluten-Free Diet." Mayo Clinic, Healthy Lifestyle: Nutrition and Healthy Eating. Mayo Clinic Staff. Accessed December 1, 2020. https://www.mayoclinic. org/healthy-lifestyle/nutrition-and-healthy-eating/in-depth/gluten-free-diet/art-20048530.

"Gluten-Free Grains." Gluten Intolerance Group. Accessed December 1, 2020. https://gluten.org/2019/10/17/gluten-free-grains/.

GMO Facts." Non-GMO Project.org. Accessed October 7, 2018. https://www.nongmoproject.org/gmo-facts/.

"Goodbye to Sugar Tooth?" The Free Library. 2000 American Dental Hygienists' Association 27 May. 2020 https://www.thefreelibrary.com/Goodbye+to+Sugar+Tooth%3f-a069291125

Gorzynik-Debicka, M., Przychodzen, P., Cappello, F., Kuban-Jankowska, A., Marino Gammazza, A., Knap, N., Wozniak, M., & Gorska-Ponikowska, M. (2018). Potential Health Benefits of Olive Oil and Plant Polyphenols. International journal of molecular sciences, 19(3), 686. https://doi.org/10.3390/ijms19030686. https://www.ncbi.nlm.nih.gov/pmc/articles/PMC5877547./

Grewal, Alison. " Differences Between Magnesium Chelates and Magnesium Citrate" Accessed October 6, 2022 Livestrong.com. https://www.livestrong.com/article/482655-differences-between-magnesium-chelate-and-magnesium-citrate/.

Griffith-Greene, Megan. "Pesticide Traces in Some Tea Exceed Allowable Limits." Canadian Broadcasting Corporation, Marketplace. Updated March 8, 2014.

https://www.cbc.ca/news/canada/pesticide-traces-in-some-tea-exceed-allowable-limits-1.2564624.

Grohol, John. "Home » Blog » Need to Form a New Habit? Give Yourself At Least 66 Days." PsychCentral.com. Accessed November 1, 2020. https://psychcentral.com/blog/need-to-form-a-new-habit-66-days/.

Groves, Melissa. "Top 12 Health Benefits of Eating Grapes." Healthline.com. August 22, 2018. https://www.healthline.com/nutrition/benefits-of-grapes.

Guenard, Rebecca. "Minimally Processed Oil." AOCS, Inform Magazine. April 2020. https://www.aocs.org/stay-informed/inform-magazine/featured-articles/minimally-processed-oils-april-2020?SSO=True.

Gunnars, Kris. "12 Proven Health Benefits of Avocado." Healthline.com. June 29, 2018. https://www.healthline.com/nutrition/12-proven-benefits-of-avocado.

Gunnars, Kris. "Xylitol: Everything You Need to Know." Healthline.com. October 4, 2018. https://www.healthline.com/nutrition/xylitol-101.

Hansen, Fawne. "Which Fruits Have the Lowest Glycemic Load?" AdrenalFatigueSolution.com. Updated October 29, 2018. https://adrenalfatiguesolution.com/fruits-lowest-glycemic-load/.

"Health Benefits of Vanilla." WebMD. Accessed January 30, 2022. https://www.webmd.com/diet/health-benefits-vanilla#1.

"Healthy Fats Reduce Diabetes Risk." Tufts University Health & Nutrition Letter. Tufts University Gerlad J. and Dorothy R. Friedman School of Nutrition Science and Policy. September 30, 2016. https://www.nutritionletter.tufts.edu/general-nutrition/healthy-fats-reduce-diabetes-risk.

"Healthy Weight." The Centers for Disease Control and Prevention. Accessed October 20, 2020. https://www.cdc.gov/diabetes/managing/healthy-weight.html.

Henry J Thompson, Mark A Brick, Perspective: Closing the Dietary Fiber Gap: An Ancient Solution for a 21st Century Problem, Advances in Nutrition, Volume 7, Issue 4, July 2016, Pages 623–626, https://doi.org/10.3945/an.115.009696.

"Herbicide Glyphosate Present in US Streams and Rivers." U.S. Geological Survey. Accessed December 11, 2020. https://www.usgs.gov/center-news/herbicide-glyphosate-prevalent-us-streams-and-rivers?qt-news_science_products=1#qt-news_science_products.

Hess-Fischl, Amy, and Lisa M. Leontis. "How to Prevent Prediabetes From Becoming Type 2 Diabetes." EndocrineWeb.com. Updated on: 07/09/19. https://www.endocrineweb.com/conditions/pre-diabetes/pre-diabetes.

Heyman, Mark. "Diabetes and Mindfulness." Taking Control of Your Diabetes, tcoyd.org. March 29, 2018. https://tcoyd.org/2018/03/diabetes-and-mindfulness/.

Hoffman JR, Falvo MJ. Protein - Which is Best?. J Sports Sci Med. 2004;3(3):118-130. Published 2004 Sep 1. https://www.ncbi.nlm.nih.gov/pmc/articles/PMC3905294/.

"How Blue Light Affects Kids and Sleep." SleepFoundation.org. Updated July 28, 2020. https://www.sleepfoundation.org/articles/how-blue-light-affects-kids-sleep.

"How Long Does it Take to Form a New Habit?" University College London, UCL News. August 4, 2009. https://www.ucl.ac.uk/news/2009/aug/how-long-does-it-take-form-habit.

"How Much Water Should I Drink? WebMD.com. Accessed November 17, 2020. https://www.webmd.com/diet/how-much-water-to-drink#1.

"How Much Water Should You Drink Every Day?" Mayo Clinic. *Healthy Lifestyle, Nutrition and Healthy Eating.* Accessed July 29, 2020. https://www.mayoclinic.org/healthy-lifestyle/nutrition-and-healthy-eating/in-depth/water/art-20044256.

"Hulled Millet" Bobsredmill.com. Accessed November 30,2020. https://www.bobsredmill.com/hulled-millet.html.

Hugues, Stacey. "Pasta Substitutes Available for People With Diabetes." VerywellHealth.com Updated March 31, 2019. https://www.verywellhealth.com/top-diabetic-pasta-substitutes-1087190.

"Hypoglycemia." Symptoms & Causes. The Mayo Clinic. Accessed December 7, 2020. https://www.mayoclinic.org/diseases-conditions/hypoglycemia/symptoms-causes/syc-20373685.

"Important Nutrients to Know: Proteins, Carbohydrates, and Fats." National Institute on Aging, National Institutes of Health. Reviewed April 29, 2019. https://www.nia.nih.gov/health/important-nutrients-know-proteins-carbohydrates-and-fats.

"Is Kamu ® t Gluten-Free?" Bobsredmill.com. Accessed November 30, 2020. https://www.bobsredmill.com/blog/healthy-living/is-kamut-gluten-free/.

Jacob, Aglaee. "How Soon After Ingestion of Food Does Blood Sugar Rise?" Healthy Eating. Sfgate.com. December 6, 2018. http://healthyeating.sfgate.com/soon-after-ingestion-food-blood-sugar-rise-1399.html.

Jacob, Aglaee. "Why Do Diabetics Need to Eat Protein With Carbs?" LiveStrong.com. Accessed May 6, 2019. https://www.livestrong.com/article/496414-why-diabetics-need-to-eat-protein-with-carbs/.

Jacob, Aglaee. "What Factors Slow the Absorption of Carbohydrates?" LiveStrong.com. Accessed May 6,

2019. https://www.livestrong.com/article/500047-what-factors-slow-the-absorption-of-carbohydrates/.

Jain R, Venkatasubramanian P. Sugarcane Molasses - A Potential Dietary Supplement in the Management of Iron Deficiency Anemia. J Diet Suppl. 2017 Sep 3;14(5):589-598. doi: 10.1080/19390211.2016.1269145. Epub 2017 Jan 26. PMID: 28125303. https://pubmed.ncbi.nlm.nih.gov/28125303/.

Jakubowicz, Daniela, Julio Wainstein, Bo Ahren, Zohar Landau, Yosefa Bar-Dayan, and Oren Froy. "Fasting Until Noon Triggers Increased Postprandial Hyperglycemia and Impaired Insulin Response After Lunch and Dinner in Individuals With Type 2 Diabetes: A Randomized Clinical Trial." Diabetes Care 38, no. 10 (October 2015): 1820-1826. http://care.diabetesjournals.org/content/38/10/1820?sid=860338a6-3135-4cc4-a97f-79b3aa292367.

Jarosh, WIllow. Malia Frey. "Almond Milk Nutrition Facts: Calories, Carbs, and Health Benefits." Verywellfit.com. February 18, 2020. https://www.verywellfit.com/almond-milk-nutrition-calories-carbs-and-benefits-4164247.

Jedha. "Agave and Diabetes: Another Nutrition Myth Busted!" DiabetesMealPlans.com. Accessed October 7, 2018. https://diabetesmealplans.com/10283/agave-and-diabetes/.

Jedha. "Lemon/Lime and Type 2 Diabetes." DiabetesMealPlans.com. Accessed October 7, 2018. https://diabetesmealplans.com/11214/lemon-lime-and-type-2-diabetes/.

Johnson, Melissa. "10 Warning Signs of Low Blood Sugar." Everyday Health.com. Updated August 28, 2017. https://www.everydayhealth.com/type-2-diabetes/symptoms/signs-of-low-blood-sugar/.

Johnson-Green, Chandra. "Stone Fruits: 8 Healthy Reasons to Keep Them Stocked." UniversityHealthNews.com. September 14, 2018. https://universityhealthnews.com/daily/nutrition/stone-fruits-8-healthy-reasons-to-keep-them-stocked/.

Juntarawijit, Chudchawal, and Yuwayong Juntarawijit. "Association Between Diabetes and Pesticides: A Case Control Study Among Thai Farmers." Environmental Health and Preventative Medicine 23, no. 3 (2018). https://environhealthprevmed.biomedcentral.com/articles/10.1186/s12199-018-0692-5.

Kahn, Alam, Mahpara Safdar, Mohammad Muzaffar Ali Khan, Khan Nawaz Khattak, and Richard A. Anderson. "Cinnamon Improves Glucose and Lipids of People With Type 2 Diabetes." Diabetes Care 26, no. 12 (December 2003: 3215-3218. http://care.diabetesjournals.org/content/26/12/3215.

Kelley DS, Adkins Y, Laugero KD. "A Review of the Health Benefits of Cherries." Nutrients. 2018;10(3):368. Published 2018 Mar 17. doi:10.3390/nu10030368

Kennedy, Kelly. Maria Masters. "8 Best Fruits for a Diabetes Friendly Diet." Everyday Health.com. September 6, 2017. https://www.everydayhealth.com/type-2-diabetes/best-fruits-for-diabetes/.

Kelly Kennedy. Mary Elizabeth Dallas. "10 Foods That Can Help With Blood Sugar Control." September 20, 2017. "September 20, 2017.

Keown, Alex, and Steve Metsch. "A Plant-Based Diet Challenge at Work Can Deliver Life-Changing Results." CommunityHealthMagazine.com. February 24, 2019. http://www.communityhealthmagazine.com/nutrition_and_fitness/a-plant-based-diet-challenge-at-work-can-deliver-life/article_116189b0-d638-11e8-a284-cb70966ae3b9.html.

Kennedy, Kelly, Katie Robinson. "Is Quinoa Good for You? Everything You Need to Know About the Superfood." EverydayHealth.com. July 8, 2019. https://www.everydayhealth.com/diet-nutrition/diet/quinoa-nutrition-facts-types-how-cook-it-more/.

Kennedy, Kelly, Stephanie Bucklin. "The Best Ways to Enjoy Dark Chocolate When You Have Diabetes." Everyday Health.com. October 17, 2017. https://www.everydayhealth.com/type-2-diabetes/diet/why-dark-chocolate-one-best-desserts-diabetics/.

Kennedy, Kelly. Margaret O'Malley. "When and How Much You Exercise Can Help Type 2 Diabetes." October 18, 2016. https://www.everydayhealth.com/type-2-diabetes/living-with/make-fitness-work-for-

you/#:~:text=In%20fact%2C%20another%2C%20
smaller%20study,better%20control%20their%20
blood%20sugar.

Kerns, Michelle. " The Glycemic Index of Applesauce." Accessed December 18, 2021. https://www.livestrong. com/article/482460-the-glycemic-index-of-applesauce/.

"Key Elements of Healthy Eating Patterns." 2015-2020 Dietary Guidelines for Americans Eighth Edition, U.S. Department of Agriculture. Accessed November 15, 2020. https://health.gov/our-work/food-nutrition/2015-2020-dietary-guidelines/guidelines/chapter-1/a-closer-look-inside-healthy-eating-patterns/#other-components.

"Know Your Blood Sugar Numbers: Use Them to Manage Your Diabetes." National Institutes of Health. March 2016. https://www.niddk.nih.gov/health-information/diabetes/overview/managing-diabetes/know-blood-sugar-numbers.

Kostoglou-Athanassiou, Ifigenia, Panagiotis Athanassiou, Anastasios Gkountouvas, and Philippos Kaldrymides. "Vitamin D and Glycemic Control in Diabetes Mellitus Type 2" Therapeutic Advances in Endocrinology and Metabolism 4, no. 4 (August 2013): 122-128. https://www.ncbi.nlm.nih.gov/pmc/articles/PMC3755528/.

Krans, Brian. "5 Blackstrap Molasses Benefits." Healthline. com. February 24, 2015. https://www.healthline.com/health/food-nutrition/benefits-blackstrap-molasses.

Krehl WA. "The Role of Nutrition in Maintaining Health and Preventing Disease." Health Values. 1983 Mar-Apr;7(2):9-13. https://www.ncbi.nlm.nih.gov/pubmed/10260843.

Krezowski PA, Nuttall FQ, Gannon MC, Bartosh NH. The effect of protein ingestion on the metabolic response to oral glucose in normal individuals. Am J Clin Nutr. 1986 Dec;44(6):847-56. doi: 10.1093/ajcn/44.6.847. PMID: 3538843.

La Magueresse-Battstoni, Brigitte, Emmanuel Labaronne, Hubert Vidal, and Danielle Naville. "Endocrine Disrupting Chemicals in Mixture and Obesity, Diabetes and Other Related Metabolic Disorders." World Journal of Biological Chemistry, 8, no. 2 (May 26, 2017): 108-119. https://www.ncbi.nlm.nih.gov/pmc/articles/PMC5439162/.

Lally, Phillippa, van Jaarsveld, C.H.M., Potts, H.W.W. and Wardle, J. First published July 16, 2019. "How are habits formed: Modeling habit formation in the real world." Eur. J. Soc. Psychol., 40: 998-1009. doi:10.1002/ejsp.674. https://onlinelibrary.wiley.com/doi/abs/10.1002/ejsp.674.

Leech, Joe. "10 Evidence-Based Health Benefits of Cinnamon." Healthline.com. July 5, 2018. https://www.healthline.com/nutrition/10-proven-benefits-of-cinnamon.

"Legumes Improve Blood Sugar Control and Reduce Cardiovascular Risk in Type 2 Diabetics." CardioSmart,

American College of Cardiology. October 26, 2012. https://www.cardiosmart.org/News-and-Events/2012/10/Legumes-improve-blood-sugar-control-and-reduce-cardiovascular-risk-in-diabetics.

Ledochowski, Larissa. Gerhard Ruedl, Adrian H. Taylor, Martin Kopp. "Acute Effects of Brisk Walking on Sugary Snack Cravings in Overweight People, Affect and Responses to a Manipulated Stress Situation and to a Sugary Snack Cue: A Crossover Study." March 11, 2015. https://journals.plos.org/plosone/article/authors?id=10.1371/journal.pone.0119278.

Leech, Joe. "10 Health Benefits of Spirulina." Healthline. com. October 5, 2018. https://www.healthline.com/nutrition/10-proven-benefits-of-spirulina#section4.

Leonard, Jayne. "Is Honey Better For You Than Sugar?" MedicalNewsToday.com. June 1, 2017. https://www.medicalnewstoday.com/articles/317728.php.

Li M, Fan Y, Zhang X, et alFruit and vegetable intake and risk of type 2 diabetes mellitus: meta-analysis of prospective cohort studiesBMJ Open 2014;4:e005497. doi: 10.1136/bmjopen-2014-005497. https://bmjopen.bmj.com/content/4/11/e005497.citation-tools.

Liles, Honah. "Sugar Can Cause Headaches, and It's More Likely if You Have Diabetes." Insider Inc. September 30, 2020. https://www.insider.com/can-sugar-cause-headache.

Lim EL, Hollingsworth KG, Aribisala BS, Chen MJ, Mathers JC, Taylor R. Reversal of type 2 diabetes: Normalisation of beta cell function in association with decreased pancreas and liver triacylglycerol. Diabetologia 2011; 54: 2506-2514. PMID 21656330

Leopold, Caroline. "Can I Eat Rice if I Have Diabetes?" MedicalNewsToday.com. Updated March 25, 2019. https://www.medicalnewstoday.com/articles/314183. php.

Leopold, Caroline. "Fruits For People With Diabetes." MedicalNewsToday.com. Updated November 19, 2018. https://www.medicalnewstoday.com/articles/311220. php.

Lewin, Jo. "The Health Benefits of Spinach." BBC, Good Food. Accessed October 20, 2020. https://www. bbcgoodfood.com/howto/guide/ingredient-focus-spinach#:~:text=Spinach%20is%20also%20an%20 excellent,in%20vitamin%20K%20than%20spinach.

"Losing Weight: What is Healthy Weight Loss?" Centers for Disease Control and Prevention. Accessed September 27, 2019. https://www.cdc.gov/ healthyweight/losing_weight/index.html.

"Low Vitamin D Levels Associated with Colds and Flu." National Institutes of Health, *NIH Research Matters*. March 2, 2009. https://www.nih.gov/news-events/ nih-research-matters/low-vitamin-d-levels-associated-colds-flu#:~:text=A%20new%20study%20has%20 found,naturally%20present%20in%20few%20foods.

Macht, Hilary. Ioanna Tzoulaki. "Common Environmental Chemicals Increase Your Risk of Diabetes." Endocrineweb.com. September 23, 2019. https://www.endocrineweb.com/news/diabetes/17611-link-between-endocrine-disrupting-chemicals-diabetes.

Mäkinen, Kauko K. "Gastrointestinal Disturbances Associated with the Consumption of Sugar Alcohols with Special Consideration of Xylitol: Scientific Review and Instructions for Dentists and Other Health-Care Professionals." International Journal of Dentistry, September 25, 2016. https://www.hindawi.com/journals/ijd/2016/5967907/.

"Magnesium Fact Sheet for Consumers." The National Institutes of Health, Office of Dietary Supplements. Updated: March 24, 2020. https://ods.od.nih.gov/factsheets/Magnesium-Consumer/#:~:text=Magnesium%20is%20a%20nutrient%20that,protein%2C%20bone%2C%20and%20DNA.

"Magnesium: Fact Sheet for Health Professionals." The National Institutes of Health. Accessed August 1, 2019. https://ods.od.nih.gov/factsheets/Magnesium-HealthProfessional/.

Mann, Madeline R. "Do's and Don'ts of Managing Diabetes When You're Sick." EverydayHealth.com. Updated March 9, 2016. https://www.everydayhealth.com/hs/type-2-diabetes-live-better-guide/sick-day-dos-donts/.

"Mannitol." Nutrients Review.com. Accessed May 6, 2019. http://www.nutrientsreview.com/carbs/sugar-alcohol-mannitol.html.

Marengo, Katherine. Aaron Kandola. "What are the Best Nuts for Diabetes?" Medical News Today.com. January 9, 2019. https://www.medicalnewstoday.com/articles/324141.php.

Marino, Mark T. "Drugs That Can Worsen Diabetes Control." DiabetesSelfManagement. com. Updated September 8, 2017. https://www.diabetesselfmanagement.com/managing-diabetes/blood-glucose-management/drugs-that-can-worsen-diabetes-control/.

Masi, L. N., Martins, A. R., Rosa Neto, J. C., do Amaral, C. L., Crisma, A. R., Vinolo, M. A., de Lima Júnior, E. A., Hirabara, S. M., & Curi, R. (2012). Sunflower oil supplementation has proinflammatory effects and does not reverse insulin resistance in obesity induced by high-fat diet in C57BL/6 mice. Journal of biomedicine & biotechnology, 2012, 945131. https://doi.org/10.1155/2012/945131

Mawer, Rudy. MSc, CISSN. "The Ketogenic Diet: A Detailed Beginner's Guide to Keto." July 30, 2018. https://www.healthline.com/nutrition/ketogenic-diet-101#types.

McCulloch, Marsha. "10 Supplements to Help Lower Blood Sugar." Healthline.com. October 29, 2018. https://www.healthline.com/nutrition/blood-sugar-supplements.

McCulloch, Marsha. "Top 13 Lean Protein Foods You Should Eat." July 15, 2018. Healthline.com https://www.healthline.com/nutrition/lean-protein-foods.

McDermott, Annette. "Monk Fruit vs. Stevia: Which Sweetener Should You Use?" Healthline.com. April 15, 2016. https://www.healthline.com/health/food-nutrition/monk-fruit-vs-stevia.

McDonell, Kayla. "Everything You Need to Know About Molasses." MedicalNewsToday.com. July 31, 2017. https://www.medicalnewstoday.com/articles/318719.php.

McKennon SA. Non-Pharmaceutical Intervention Options for Type 2 Diabetes: Diets and Dietary Supplements (Botanicals, Antioxidants, and Minerals) [Updated 2018 Jun 18]. In: Feingold KR, Anawalt B, Boyce A, et al., editors. Endotext [Internet]. South Dartmouth (MA): MDText.com, Inc.; 2000-. Available from: https://www.ncbi.nlm.nih.gov/books/NBK279062

"Meditation: A Simple, Fast Way to Reduce Stress." The Mayo Clinic, Health Information. Accessed December 22, 2020. https://www.mayoclinic.org/tests-procedures/meditation/in-depth/meditation/art-20045858.

"Metformin and Vitamin B12 Deficiency." Life Extension Magazine, August 2007. https://www.lifeextension.

Mignone, L. E., Wu, T., Horowitz, M., & Rayner, C. K. (2015). Whey protein: The "whey" forward for treatment of type 2 diabetes?. World journal of diabetes, 6(14), 1274–1284. https://doi.org/10.4239/wjd.v6.i14.1274.

"Millet Flour." Bobsredmill. Accessed November 30, 2020. https://www.bobsredmill.com/millet-flour.html.

Mirmiran, P., Houshialsadat, Z., Gaeini, Z., Bahadoran, Z., & Azizi, F. (2020). Functional properties of beetroot (Beta vulgaris) in management of cardio-metabolic diseases. Nutrition & metabolism, 17, 3. https://doi.org/10.1186/s12986-019-0421-0 com/magazine/2007/8/atp/page-01?p=1.

Miller, Carla K. "Jean L. Kristeller, Amy Headings, Haikady Nagaraja, W. Fred Miser. Comparative Effectiveness of a Mindful Eating Intervention to a Diabetes Self-Management Intervention among Adults with Type 2 Diabetes: A Pilot Study. Journal of the Academy of Nutrition and Dietetics, 2012; 112 (11): 1835 DOI: 10.1016/j.jand.2012.07.036.

Miller, K. B., Hurst, W. J., Payne, M. J., Stuart, D. A., Apgar, J., Sweigart, D. S., & Ou, B. (2008). Impact of alkalization on the antioxidant and flavanol content of commercial cocoa powders. Journal of agricultural and food chemistry, 56(18), 8527–8533.

Monro, John A. (2013) "Kiwifruit, Carbohydrate Availability, and the Glycemic Response." Advances in Food and Nutrition Research 68, February 5, 2013.

https://www.sciencedirect.com/science/article/pii/
B9780123942944000146?via%3Dihub.

Morais JBS1, Severo JS1, de Alencar GRR1, de Oliveira
ARS1, Cruz KJC1, Marreiro DDN1, Freitas BJESA1,
de Carvalho CMR1, Martins MDCCE2, Frota
KMG3. Nutrition. 2017 Jun;38:54-60. doi: 10.1016/j.
nut.2017.01.009. Epub 2017 Feb 2. "Effect of
magnesium supplementation on insulin resistance in
humans: A systematic review." https://www.ncbi.nlm.
nih.gov/pubmed/28526383.

Nayak, Prathibha Anand, Ullal Anand Nayak, and Vishal
Khandelwal. Clinical, Cosmetic and Investigational
Dentistry, no. 6 (November 10, 2014): 89-94. "The
Effect of Xylitol on Dental Caries and Dental Flora."
https://www.dovepress.com/the-effect-of-xylitol-on-
dental-caries-and-oral-flora-peer-reviewed-article-
CCIDE.

Neithercott, Tracey. "Cooking With Oils,"
DiabetesForecast.org. March 2011. http://www.
diabetesforecast.org/2011/mar/cooking-with-oils.html.

Neithercott, Tracey. "The Art of Grazing."
DiabetesForecast.org. October 2008. http://www.
diabetesforecast.org/2008/oct/the-art-of-grazing.html.

"Newcastle Study: 600 Calorie Diet." Diabetes.co.uk.
March 1, 2019. https://www.diabetes.co.uk/diet/
newcastle-study-600-calorie-diet.html.

"New Research Finds Artificial Sweeteners Can Cause Type 2 Diabetes." Medical College of Wisconsin, *Newsroom*. October 8, 2018. https://www.mcw.edu/ newsroom/news-articles/new-research-finds-artificial-sweeteners-can-cause-type-2-diabetes.

"Type 2 Diabetes is a Reversible Condition." ScienceDaily. www.sciencedaily.com/ releases/2017/09/170913084432.htm (accessed November 4, 2020).

"Non-Starchy Vegetables." American Diabetes Association. Updated August 25, 2017. http://www.diabetes.org/ food-and-fitness/food/what-can-i-eat/making-healthy-food-choices/non-starchy-vegetables.html.

Nordqvist, Christian "All About Hypoglycemia (Low Blood Sugar)." MedicalNewsToday.com. Updated March 11, 2019. https://www.medicalnewstoday.com/ articles/166815.php.

Nordqvist, Joseph. "What are the Benefits and Risks of Whey Protein?" MedicalNewsToday.com. Updated November 27, 2017. https://www.medicalnewstoday. com/articles/263371.php.

"Nutrition Management of Low Blood Sugar Without Diabetes" (Postprandial Syndrome and Reactive Hypoglycemia). University of Wisconsin Hospitals, UW Health, Health Facts For You. Accessed June 21, 2020. https://www.uwhealth.org/healthfacts/ nutrition/396.pdf.

"Nuts and Your Heart. Eating Nuts for Heart Health." Mayo Clinic. Accessed June 24, 2019. https://www.mayoclinic.org/diseases-conditions/heart-disease/in-depth/nuts/art-20046635.

"Nuts for the Heart." T.H. Chan School of Public Health Nutrition Source. Accessed January 17, 2020. https://www.hsph..edu/nutritionsource/nuts-for-the-heart/.

O'Malley, Margaret. "5 Sugar Substitutes for Type 2 Diabetes." EverydayHealth.com. Accessed May 6, 2019. https://www.everydayhealth.com/type-2-diabetes/diet/sugar-substitutes-for-diabetes/.

Oberst, Lindsay. "Xylitol vs. Erythritol: Which is the Healthier Sugar Substitute?" Healthline.com. July 31, 2017. https://www.healthline.com/health/food-nutrition/xylitol-vs-erythritol#1.

Ohio State University. "Cholesterol Medication Could invite Diabetes, Study Suggests: Patient data shows association between statins and type 2 diabetes." ScienceDaily. www.sciencedaily.com/releases/2019/06/190625102434.htm (accessed June 18, 2020).

Olsen, Natalie. Cathleen Crichton-Stuart. "Can People With Diabetes Eat Potatoes?" Medical News Today.com. May 13, 2019. https://www.medicalnewstoday.com/articles/323449.php#potatoes-and-diabetes.

Olsen, Natalie. Brian Krans. "How Wheat Germ Benefits Your Health." September 17, 2018. https://www. healthline.com/health/wheat-germ-benefits#1., Natalie. Zawn Villines. "Top 15 Sources of Plant-Based Protein." April 12, 2018. https://www. medicalnewstoday.com/articles/321474.

"Organic Kamut®" Berries. Bobsredmill.com. Accessed November 30, 2020. https://www.bobsredmill.com/ organic-Kamut-berries.html.

Orlov, Alex. "The Real Scoop: Frozen Yogurt Only Sounds Healthier Than Ice Cream." CNN.com. August 10, 2015. https://www.cnn.com/2015/07/27/health/frozen-yogurt-versus-ice-cream/index.html.

Palinski-Wade, Erin. "5 Surprising Foods That Have Little Impact on Blood Sugar" EverydayHealth. com. Accessed November 23, 2018. https://www. everydayhealth.com/pictures/surprising-foods-little-impact-blood-sugar/#02.

Pallarito, Karen. "15 Ways High Blood Sugar Affects Your Body." Health.com. Updated December 17, 2018. https://www.health.com/type-2-diabetes/high-blood-sugar-symptoms.

Panzarella, Anna. "5 Ways to Stabilize Blood Sugar With Meal Timing." WebMD.com. https://blogs.webmd. com/diabetes/20160621/5-ways-to-stabilize-blood-sugar-with-meal-timing.

"Peaches, Plums, Nectarines Give Obesity, Diabetes Slim Chance." ScienceDaily.com. June 18, 2012. https://www.sciencedaily.com/releases/2012/06/120618132921.htm.

"Pears and Diabetes." USAPears.org. Accessed October 7, 2018. Retrieved from https://usapears.org/pears-and-diabetes/.

People with Prediabetes Who Drop Substantial Weight May Ward Off Type 2 Diabetes." Johns Hopkins Medicine. July 16, 2013. https://www.hopkinsmedicine.org/news/media/releases/people_with_pre_diabetes_who_drop_substantial_weight_may_ward_off_type_2_diabetes.

Pérez-Guisado, Joaquín, and Andrés Muñoz-Serrano. "A Pilot Study of the Spanish Ketogenic Mediterranean Diet: An Effective Therapy for the Metabolic Syndrome." Journal of Medicinal Food 14, no. 7-8: July 15, 2011. https://www.liebertpub.com/doi/10.1089/jmf.2010.0137.

Peters, Brandon. "How Screen Light From Devices Affects Your Sleep." VerywellHealth.com Updated October 28, 2018. https://www.verywellhealth.com/how-does-screen-light-affect-sleep-3014732.

"Pesticides." Diabetesandenvironment.org. Accessed January 20, 2019. http://www.diabetesandenvironment.org/home/contam/pesticides.

Pflipsen, Matthew C., Robert C. Oh, Aaron Saguil, Dean A. Seehusen, Derek Seaquist, and Richard Topolski. "The Prevalence of Vitamin B12 Deficiency in Patients With Type 2 Diabetes: A Cross-Sectional Study." Journal of the American Board of Family Medicine 22, no. 5 (September-October 2009): 528-534. https://www.jabfm.org/content/22/5/528.

Peggy Pletcher. Mandy Ferreira. "Seven Health Benefits of Coconut Water." Medical News Today.com. July 12, 2017. https://www.medicalnewstoday.com/articles/318394#:~:text=Coconut%20water%20is%20made%20from,of%20coconut%20water%20is%20water.

Pletcher, Peggy. Roland, James. "How Does Eating Affect Your Blood Sugar?" Healthline.com. January 4, 2017. Updated January 2, 2020. https://www.healthline.com/health/and-after-effect-eating-blood-sugar.

"Prediabetes." The Mayo Clinic. Accessed November 1, 2020. https://www.mayoclinic.org/diseases-conditions/prediabetes/symptoms-causes/syc-20355278.

"Prediabetes." Diagnosis & Treatment. The Mayo Clinic. Accessed December 7, 2020. https://www.mayoclinic.org/diseases-conditions/prediabetes/diagnosis-treatment/drc-20355284.

"Prediabetes. What is it?" Medical School. Health Publishing. December 2018. "https://www.health..edu/a_to_z/pre-diabetes-a-to-z."

Prelipcean, Maria, Claire Sissons. "Can Eating Too Much Fruit Cause Type 2 Diabetes?" Medical News Today. com. April 26, 2019. https://www.medicalnewstoday. com/articles/323310.

"Prevent Type 2 Diabetes." The Centers for Disease Control and Prevention." Accessed October 20, 2020. https:// www.cdc.gov/diabetes/pdfs/library/socialmedia/HCP-infographic.pdf?s_cid=cs_5164 .

"Preventing Type 2 Diabetes." NIH National Institute of Diabetes and Digestive and Kidney Diseases. December 2016. https://www.niddk.nih.gov/health-information/diabetes/overview/preventing-type-2-diabetes.

"Protein." T.H. Chan School of Public Health, *Nutrition Source*. Accessed December 1, 2020. https://www. hsph..edu/nutritionsource/what-should-you-eat/protein/.

Raymond, Joan. "Can You Stop Diabetes Meds?" WebMD. com. Reviewed May 3, 2016. https://www.webmd.com/diabetes/features/stop-diabetes-meds-doctor#1.

Rena R. Wing, Wei Lang, Thomas A. Wadden, Monika Safford, William C. Knowler, Alain G. Bertoni, James O. Hill, Frederick L. Brancati, Anne Peters, Lynne Wagenknecht, the Look AHEAD Research Group. " Benefits of Modest Weight Loss in Improving Cardiovascular Risk Factors in Overweight and Obese Individuals With Type 2 Diabetes." *Diabetes Care*. July 2011. https://care.diabetesjournals.org/

content/34/7/1481.full.

"Research spotlight - Putting Type 2 Diabetes Into Remission." Reviewed June 28, 2019. https://www. diabetes.org.uk/research/research-round-up/research-spotlight/research-spotlight-low-calorie-liquid-diet.

Ricciotti, Hope. Toni Golden. "Can I Reverse Prediabetes?" Medical School. Health Publishing. Women's Health Watch. November, 2019. https://www.health..edu/ diseases-and-conditions/can-i-reverse-prediabetes.

Riddell, M., & Perkins, B. A. (2009). Exercise and glucose metabolism in persons with diabetes mellitus: perspectives on the role for continuous glucose monitoring. Journal of diabetes science and technology, 3(4), 914–923. https://doi. org/10.1177/193229680900300439

Riddle, Jim (2012, July 5) "Organic Dairy Certification: Why, How, and What?" Cooperative Extension System. July 5, 2012. http://articles.extension.org/pages/18336/ organic-dairy-certification:-why-how-and-what.

Roussel R, Fezeu L, Bouby N, et al. "Low Water Intake and Risk for New-Onset Hyperglycemia." Accessed July 25, 2020. Diabetes Care. 2011;34(12):2551-2554. doi:10.2337/dc11-0652 . https://pubmed.ncbi.nlm.nih. gov/21994426/.

Sakimura, Johannah. "10 Surprising Causes of Blood Sugar Swings You Probably Didn't Know." EverydayHealth.

com. Updated September 18, 2017. https://www.
everydayhealth.com/type-2-diabetes/symptoms/
surprising-causes-of-blood-sugar-swings/.

Salas-Salvadó, Jordi, et al. "Reduction in the Incidence
of Type 2 Diabetes With the Mediterranean Diet."
Diabetes Care 34, no. 1 (January 2011): 14-19. http://
care.diabetesjournals.org/content/34/1/14.

Salkeld, Lauren. "Freeze Kale for Quick Smoothies and
Last-Minute Meals." Eatingwell.com. April 14, 2020.
https://www.eatingwell.com/article/7775702/freeze-
kale/.

Saplakoglu, Yasemin. "Scientists Warn BPA-Free Plastic
May Not Be Safe."Livescience.com September 15, 2018.
https://www.livescience.com/63592-bpa-free-plastic-
dangers.html.

Sboros, Marika. "Can You 'Cure' Type 2 Diabetes With
Diet? Just Ask Dr. Jay Wortman" Biznews.com,
February 27, 2015. https://www.biznews.com/health/
low carb-healthy-fat-science/2015/02/27/can-you-
cure-type-2-diabetes-with-diet-dr-jay-wortman-
proves-you-can.

Shan, Z., Rehm, C. D., Rogers, G., Ruan, M., Wang, D. D.,
Hu, F. B., Mozaffarian, D., Zhang, F. F., & Bhupathiraju,
S. N. (2019). Trends in Dietary Carbohydrate, Protein,
and Fat Intake and Diet Quality Among US Adults,
1999-2016. JAMA, 322(12), 1178–1187. https://doi.
org/10.1001/jama.2019.13771.

Schuna, Carly. "Pea Protein vs. Whey Protein." Livestrong. com. Accessed May 6, 2019. https://www.livestrong. com/article/281176-pea-protein-vs-whey-protein/.

Schwader, Ashley. "Benefits of Greek Yogurt." Livestrong. com. Accessed January 17, 2020. https://www. livestrong.com/article/86488-benefits-greek-yogurt/

"Severe Hypoglycemia." Diabetes.co.uk. January 15, 2019. https://www.diabetes.co.uk/severe-hypoglycemia.html.

Sherman, James R. Quote on page 163. This quote and similar versions are often attributed to James R. Sherman. Accessed November 2018. https:// quoteinvestigator.com/2015/11/05/new-ending/.

Shah Murad, Dureshehwar Marwat, Shahina, et al. "Diabetes Mellitus can be Treated and Prevented by Figs", International Journal of Research in Pharmacy and Biosciences, vol. 6, no. 2.pp. 33-36, 2019. http:// www.ijrpb.org/papers/v6-i2/5.pdf.'

"Should You Work Chocolate into Your Diet?" Health Publishing, Medical School. May 2015. https:// www.health..edu/staying-healthy/should-you-work-chocolate-into-your-diet.

"Should Dogs Eat Peanut Butter?" ASPCA Insurance. Accessed December 5, 2020. https://www. aspcapetinsurance.com/peanut-butter-month/.

Should You Try the Keto Diet?" Medical School, *health Publishing*. Accessed October 24, 2020. https://www.health..edu/staying-healthy/should-you-try-the-keto-diet.

"Short Sleep Duration Among US Adults." Centers for Disease Control and Prevention, Sleep and Sleep Disorders, Data and Statistics. Accessed September 9, 2020. https://www.cdc.gov/sleep/data_statistics.html.

Shukla, Alpana P., Radu G. Iliescu, Catherine E. Thomas, and Louis J. Aronne. "Food Order Has a Significant Impact on Postprandial Glucose and Insulin Levels." Diabetes Care. 0.2337/dc15-0429 https://care.diabetesjournals.org/content/38/7/e98?sid=ea6d4bd4-98f6-4347-9238-15e2a4c019db.

Shyamala, B.N., M. Madhava Naidu, G. Sulochanamma, and P. Srinivas. "Studies on the Antioxidant Activities of Natural Vanilla Extract and Its Constituents Through In Vitro Models." Journal of Agricultural and Food Chemistry, 55, no. 19 (August 2007): 7738-7743. https://pubs.acs.org/doi/10.1021/jf071349%2B.

Sifferlin, Alexandra. "The Ten Best and Worst Oils for Your Health." Time Magazine, Health, Diet Nutrition. July 23, 2018. https://time.com/5342337/best-worst-cooking-oils-for-your-health/.

Skerrett, Patrick. "Vitamin B12 Deficiency Can Be Sneaky, Harmful." Health Blog (blog), Health Publishing, Medical School, *Health Blog*. Updated February 11, 2019. https://www.health..edu/blog/vitamin-b12-

deficiency-can-be-sneaky-harmful-201301105780.

Sleiman D, Al-Badri MR, Azar ST. Effect of Mediterranean Diet in Diabetes Control and Cardiovascular Risk Modification: A Systematic Review. Front Public Health. 2015;3:69. Published 2015 Apr 28. doi:10.3389/fpubh.2015.00069.

Singh, C. K., Liu, X., & Ahmad, N. (2015). Resveratrol, in its natural combination in whole grape, for health promotion and disease management. Annals of the New York Academy of Sciences, 1348(1), 150–160. https://doi.org/10.1111/nyas.12798.

Sollid, Kris. "What is Xylitol?" Food Insight.org. January 3, 2019. https://foodinsight.org/what-is-xylitol/.

Spenser, Ben. "A Cure for Diabetes: Crash Diet Can Reverse Type 2 in Three Months...and Isobel and Tony are Living Proof That You CAN Stop This Killer Disease." Published December 5, 2017, Updated: December 6, 2017. https://www.dailymail.co.uk/health/article-5149557/Three-month-diet-reverse-Type-2-diabetes.html.

Spero, David. "Diabetes: Good, Bad, or What?" DiabetesSelfManagement.com. February 12, 2014. https://www.diabetesselfmanagement.com/blog/soy-and-diabetes-good-bad-or-what/.

Spero, David. "Healthy Fats for Diabetes?" DiabetesSelfManagement.com June 25, 2018. https://

www.diabetesselfmanagement.com/blog/healthy-fats-for-diabetes/.

Staughton, John. "7 Amazing Benefits of Safflower Oil." OrganicFacts.net. March 8, 2019. https://www.organicfacts.net/health-benefits/oils/safflower-oil.html.

"Steel Cut Oats vs. Rolled Oats." Nuts.com. Accessed September1, 2020. https://nuts.com/healthy-eating/steel cut-vs-rolled-oats#:~:text=Steel%20cuts%20oats%20have%20a,Taste%20and%20texture.

Stull, April J, Dorothy Klimis-Zacas, ed. "Blueberries' Impact on Insulin Resistance and Glucose Intolerance." Special issue, Antioxidants: Berry Antioxidants in Health and Disease 5, no. 4 (November 29, 2016): 44. https://www.ncbi.nlm.nih.gov/pmc/articles/PMC5187542/.

"Strawberries May Benefit People with Diabetes." EverydayHealth.com. Updated November 14, 2017. https://www.everydayhealth.com/diabetes/strawberries-may-benefit-people-with-diabetes/.

Sugar Alcohols." US Food and Drug Administration. Accessed May 6, 2019. https://www.accessdata.fda.gov/scripts/InteractiveNutritionFactsLabel/sugar-alcohol.html.

"Sugar Alcohols Fact Sheet." Interactive Nutrition Facts Label. USFDA US Food and Drug Administration. Accessed December 3, 2020. https://www.accessdata.

fda.gov/scripts/InteractiveNutritionFactsLabel/sugar-alcohols.cfm.

Sullivan, Debra. "Bromelain." Healthline.com. April 21, 2020. https://www.healthline.com/health/bromelain.

Suny Downstate Medical Center. "Low carb Diet Reduces Inflammation And Blood Saturated Fat In Metabolic Syndrome." Accessed January 15, 2021.ScienceDaily. www.sciencedaily.com/releases/2007/12/071203091236.htm.

Syn, Mia. Malia Frey. "Coconut Milk Nutrition Facts. Coconut Milk Calories, Carbs, and Health Benefits" Verywellfit.com. January 23, 2020. https://www.verywellfit.com/coconut-milk-nutrition-facts-calories-and-health-benefits-4110358.

Tan, Xiao, Lieve van Egmond, Colin D. Chapman, Jonathan Cedernaes, and Christian Benedict. "Aiding Sleep in Type 2 Diabetes: Therapeutic Considerations." The Lancet 6, no. 1 (January 1, 2018): 60-68. https://www.thelancet.com/journals/landia/article/PIIS2213-8587(17)30233-4/fulltext.

Taylor, Roy. "Reversing Type 2 Diabetes" Research. Newcastle University's Findings Could Benefit Millions of People Across the Globe." Newcastle University Research. Accessed November 1, 2020. https://www.ncl.ac.uk/research/impact/casestudies/diabetes/.

Taylor, Roy. Ahmad AI-Mrabeh, Sviatlana Zhyzhneuskaya, John C. Mathers, Naveed Sattar, Michael E.J. Lean. " Remission of Human Type 2 Diabetes Requires Decrease in Liver and Pancreas Fat Content but Is Dependent upon Capacity for J3 Cell Recovery." October 2, 2018, Cell Metabolism 28, 547-556. https:/ /doi.org/10.1 016/j.cmet.2018.07.003. https://www.ncl.ac.uk/media/wwwnclacuk/ newcastlemagneticresonancecentre/files/Taylor%20 et%20al%20Cell%20Metabolism%202018.pdf,

Tello, Monique. "Healthy Lifestyle Healthy Can Prevent Diabetes (and Even Reverse It)." Health Publishing, Medical School, *Health Blog.* September 5, 2018. https://www.health..edu/blog/healthy-lifestyle-can-prevent-diabetes-and-even-reverse-it-2018090514698.

"The Big Picture: Checking Your Blood Glucose." The American Diabetes Association. Accessed July 20, 2020. https://www.diabetes.org/diabetes/medication-management/blood-glucose-testing-and-control/ checking-your-blood-glucose. Reprinted with permission The American Diabetes Association. Copyright 2020 by the American Diabetes Association.

"The Glycemic Index." Nutrition Data. Accessed January 8, 2021. https://nutritiondata.self.com/topics/ glycemic-index.

"The Glycemic Index of Sweet Corn." The University of Sydney. Accessed January 14, 2019. http://glycemicindex.com/foodSearch.

php?num=78&ak=detail.

"The Liver and Blood Sugar." Diabetes Education Online. Diabetes Teaching Center at the University of California, San Francisco. Accessed on March 21, 2020. https://dtc.ucsf.edu/types-of-diabetes/type1/ understanding-type-1-diabetes/how-the-body-processes-sugar/the-liver-blood-sugar/

"The Lowdown on Glycemic Index and Glycemic Load." Health Publishing, Medical School *Healthbeat* (blog). Accessed January 16, 2020. https://www.health..edu/ diseases-and-conditions/the-lowdown-on-glycemic-index-and-glycemic-load.

Torborg, Liza. "Mayo Clinic Q and A: How Much Vitamin D Do I Need?" Mayo Clinic. April 25, 2017. https://newsnetwork.mayoclinic.org/discussion/ mayo-clinic-q-and-a-how-much-vitamin-d-do-i-need/.

Trichopoulou, Antonia, et al. "Definitions and Potential Health Benefits of the Mediterranean Diet: Views from Experts Around the World." BMC Medicine 12, no. 112 (July 24, 2014). https://bmcmedicine.biomedcentral.com/ articles/10.1186/1741-7015-12-112.

Tremblay, Sylvie. "Apricots & Blood Sugar." SFGate.com. Updated November 21, 2018. https://healthyeating. sfgate.com/apricots-blood-sugar-9889.html.

"The Leading Countries in Vanilla Production in The World." Economics, Worldatlas.com. Accessed December 31, 2018. https://www.worldatlas.com/ articles/the-leading-countries-in-vanilla-production-in-the-world.html.

"The Sugar-Free Substance Xylitol is Poison for Dogs." DrJustineLee.com, Animal Safety (blog). Accessed January 21, 2019. https://drjustinelee.com/sugar-free-substance-xylitol-poison-dogs/.

"The Truth About Non-Fermented vs. Fermented Soy Protein" Fitday.com. Accessed October 7, 2018. https://www.fitday.com/fitness-articles/nutrition/ healthy-eating/the-truth-about-non-fermented-vs-fermented-soy-protein.html.

Tsaban, Gal. Anat Yaskolka Meir,Ehud Rinott,Hila Zelicha,Alon Kaplan,Aryeh Shalev,Amos Katz,Assaf Rudich,Amir Tirosh,Ilan Shelef,Ilan Youngster,Sharon Lebovitz,Noa Israeli,May Shabat,Dov Brikner,Efrat Pupkin,Michael Stumvoll,Joachim Thiery,Uta Ceglarek,John T Heiker,Antje Körner,Kathrin.

Landgraf,Martin von Bergen,Matthias Blüher,Meir J Stampfer, Iris Shai "The Effect of Green Mediterranean Diet on Cardiometabolic Risk; A Randomised Controlled Trial." *Heart.* November 25, 2020. https://heart.bmj.com/content/ early/2020/11/25/heartjnl-2020-317802.

Tsi, Allison. "Why You Need to Get More Sleep." Diabetes Forecast. July 2016. http://www.diabetesforecast.

org/2016/jul-aug/sleep.html#targetText=But%20
for%20people%20with%20diabetes,risk%20for%20
type%202%20diabetes.

"Types of Fats." The T.H. Chan School of Public Health,
The Nutrition Source. Accessed September 7, 2020.
https://www.hsph..edu/nutritionsource/what-should-
you-eat/fats-and-cholesterol/types-of-fat/.

"Two Small Studies Indicate Benefits of Whey Protein
for Type 2 Diabetes Control."Diabetes,co.uk. March
9, 2017. https://www.diabetes.co.uk/news/2017/mar/
two-small-studies-indicate-benefits-of-whey-protein-
for-type-2-diabetes-control-94525480.html.

Ulrika Ericson, Sophie Hellstrand, Louise Brunkwall,
Christina-Alexandra Schulz, Emily Sonestedt, Peter
Wallström, Bo Gullberg, Elisabet Wirfält, Marju
Orho-Melander, Food sources of fat may clarify the
inconsistent role of dietary fat intake for incidence
of type 2 diabetes, The American Journal of Clinical
Nutrition, Volume 101, Issue 5, May 2015, Pages
1065–1080, https://doi.org/10.3945/ajcn.114.103010.

Upton, Julie. "10 Surprising Facts About Cherries. *The
summertime favorite packs myriad health benefits.*"
US News and World Report. June 7, 2016. https://
health.usnews.com/health-news/blogs/eat-run/
articles/2016-06-07/10-surprising-facts-about-
cherries#:~:text=Cherries%20have%20among%20
the%20lowest,to%2055%20is%20considered%20low.

Upton, Julie. "Is Dairy-Free Ice Cream Actually Better For You?" Health.com. Updated September 14, 2018. https://www.health.com/nutrition/dairy-free-ice-cream-healthy.

Urban JD, Carakostas MC, Taylor SL. Steviol glycoside safety: are highly purified steviol glycoside sweeteners food allergens? Food Chem Toxicol. 2015 Jan;75:71-8. doi: 10.1016/j.fct.2014.11.011. Epub 2014 Nov 18. PMID: 25449199.

US Department of Agriculture: Agriculture Marketing Services, "Organic Standards." Accessed November 6, 2019. https://www.ams.usda.gov/grades-standards/organic-standards.

USDHH National Institutes of Health: National Institute of Diabetes and Digestive and Kidney Diseases. "What is Diabetes?" Accessed October 7, 2018. https://www.niddk.nih.gov/health-information/diabetes/overview/what-is-diabetes.

Valente, Lisa. "Clean-Eating Foods List." EatingWell.com. Accessed October 7, 2018. http://www.eatingwell.com/article/282469/clean-eating-foods-list/.

Van Bruggen A.H.C., He M.M., Shin K., Mai V., Jeong K.C, Finckh M.R., MorrisJ.G.Jr., "Science of the Total Environment." Volumes 616–617, March 2018, Pages 255-268. https://www.sciencedirect.com/science/article/pii/S0048969717330279.

Van Dam, Rob M., Wilrike J. Pasman, Petra Verhoef. "Effects of Coffee Consumption on Fasting Blood Glucose and Insulin Concentrations." Diabetes Care. Accessed December 1, 2020. https://care. diabetesjournals.org/content/27/12/2990.

"Vanilla Patch Cures Sweet Tooth." BBC News, *Health*. July, 2000. http://news.bbc.co.uk/2/hi/health/848621. stm.

Villines, Zawn. "Cinnamon, Blood Sugar, and Diabetes." MedicalNewsToday.com. Updated April 23, 2019. https://www.medicalnewstoday.com/articles/317207. php.

Vinoy, S., Laville, M., & Feskens, E. J. (2016). Slow-release carbohydrates: growing evidence on metabolic responses and public health interest. Summary of the symposium held at the 12th European Nutrition Conference (FENS 2015). Food & nutrition research, 60, 31662. https://doi.org/10.3402/fnr.v60.31662.

"Vitamin B12: Fact Sheet for Health Professionals." National Institutes of Health: Office of Dietary Supplements. Accessed November 12, 2018. https://ods.od.nih.gov/factsheets/VitaminB12-HealthProfessional.

"Vitamin B12." Mayo Clinic. Accessed October 17, 2020. https://www.mayoclinic.org/drugs-supplements-vitamin-b12/art-20363663.

"Vitamin C Found to Help Type 2 Diabetes." Diabetes NSW and ACT. February 11, 2019. https://diabetesnsw.com.au/helpful-resources/news/vitamin-c-found-to-help-type-2/.

"Vitamin C" NIH, U.S. National Library of Medicine, *Medicine Plus.* Accessed October 20, 2020. https://medlineplus.gov/ency/article/002404.htm.

"Vitamin D: Fact Sheet for Health Professionals." National Institutes of Health: Office of Dietary Supplements. Accessed November 23, 2018. https://ods.od.nih.gov/factsheets/VitaminD-HealthProfessional/.

"Vitamin D and Health" T.H. Chan School of Public Health *Nutrition Source.* Accessed January 18, 2019. https://www.hsph..edu/nutritionsource/what-should-you-eat/vitamins/vitamin-d/.

Wake Forest University. "Daily dose of beet juice promotes brain health in older adults." ScienceDaily. Accessed October 12, 2020. www.sciencedaily.com/releases/2010/11/101102130957.htm.

Waldman, Lindsey. Barbie Cervoni. "An Overview of Eating Fruit When You Have Diabetes." November 02, 2019. https://www.verywellhealth.com/fruits-to-avoid-if-you-have-diabetes-1087587.

"Walnuts are the Healthiest Nut, Say Scientists." BBC News.com, Health. March 28, 2011. http://www.bbc.com/news/health-12865291.

Ware, Megan. "What are the Health Benefits of Kale?" MedicalNewsToday.com. Updated September 25, 2017. https://www.medicalnewstoday.com/articles/270435.php.

Warwick, Kathy. Jerisha Parker Gordon. "Can I Eat Watermelon if I Have Diabetes," Healthline.com. Updated April 17, 2020. https://www.healthline.com/health/diabetes/watermelon-and-diabetes.

Warwick, Kathy. Megan Ware. "What to Know About Cranberries." Medical News Today.com. November 1, 2019. https://www.medicalnewstoday.com/articles/269142#risks.

"Water and Diabetes." January 15, 2019. Diabetes.co.uk. https://www.diabetes.co.uk/food/water-and-diabetes.html.

Weatherspoon, Deborah. Zawn Villines, " How to Test for Diabetes at Home" Medical News Today.com. April 23, 2019. Zawn Villines. on April 23, 2019. https://www.medicalnewstoday.com/articles/317224#interpreting-results.

Wei-Haas, Maya. "Why BPA-free May Not Mean a Plastic Product is Safe." Accessed April 27, 2020. National Geographic.con. https://www.nationalgeographic.com/science/2018/09/news-BPA-free-plastic-safety-chemicals-health/.

Weiller, Claude S. "What Does 'First Cold Pressed' Olive Oil Really Mean?" CaliforniaOliveRanch.com. September 8, 2009. https://californiaoliveranch.com/what-does-first-cold-pressed-olive-olive-oil-really-mean/.

Westphalen, Dena. Jennifer Huizen. "Can You Eat Grapefruit While Taking Metformin?" Medical News Today.com. November 7, 2018. https://www.medicalnewstoday.com/articles/323603.php.

West, Helen. "9 Signs and Symptoms of Vitamin B12 Deficiency." Healthline.com. October 7, 2017. https://www.healthline.com/nutrition/vitamin-b12-deficiency-symptoms.

"What Does Extra Virgin Mean?" The California Olive Oil Council. Accessed October 3, 2019. https://www.cooc.com/what-does-extra-virgin-mean/.

"What is An Ancient Grain?" Oldways Whole Grains Council. Accessed November 1, 2020. https://wholegrainscouncil.org/whole grains-101/whats-whole grain/ancient-grains.

"What is BPA, And What Are The Concerns About BPA?" Mayo Clinic, Nutrition and Healthy Eating. Accessed November 1, 2020. https://www.mayoclinic.org/healthy-lifestyle/nutrition-and-healthy-eating/expert-answers/bpa/faq-20058331#:~:text=Some%20research%20has%20shown%20that,can%20also%20affect%20children's%20behavior.

"What Medicines Can Make Your Blood Sugar Spike?"
WedMD.com. Reviewed March 17, 2017. https://
www.webmd.com/diabetes/medicines-blood-sugar-
spike.

"What Potatoes Have the Highest Glycemic Index?"
(2016, July). Health & Nutrition Letter, Tufts
University Friedman School of Nutrition Science and
Policy: Ask Tufts Experts. January 2016. https://www.
nutritionletter.tufts.edu/issues/12_1/ask-experts/Q-
I-keep-reading-that-potatoes-are-high glycemic-
index_1860-1.html.

"Wheat Berries." Eatwheat.org. Accessed December 1,
2020. https://eatwheat.org/learn/wheat-berries/.

"Wheat Germ." Bobsredmill.com Accessed December
1, 2020. https://www.bobsredmill.com/wheat-germ.
html.

"White, brown, raw, honey: which type of sugar is best?"
21 March, 2018. SBS.com, Food. https://www.sbs.com.
au/food/article/2018/03/21/white-brown-raw-honey-
which-type-sugar-best.

"Whole Grains." The Nutrition Source, T.H. Chan School
of Public Health. Accessed October 7, 2018. https://
www.hsph..edu/nutritionsource/whole grains/.

"Whole Grains A to Z." Oldways Whole Grains
Council. Accessed November 2, 2020. https://
wholegrainscouncil.org/whole grains-101/whole

grains-z#teff.

"WHO Calls on Countries to Reduce Sugars Intake Among Adults and Children." World Health Organization. March 4, 2015. https://www.who.int/news/item/04-03-2015-who-calls-on-countries-to-reduce-sugars-intake-among-adults-and-children.

"Why Fiber Is So Good For You." The University of Southern California, UCSF Benioff Children's Hospital. Accessed January 17, 2020. https://www.ucsfbenioffchildrens.org/education/why_fiber_is_so_good_for_you/.

"Why Monk Fruit is A Power Food for Diabetes." The Diabetes Council team. Accessed November 2, 2020. https://www.thediabetescouncil.com/why-monk-fruit-is-a-power-food-for-diabetes/.

"Why Zero-Calorie Sweeteners Can Still Lead to Diabetes, Obesity: Common Artificial Sweeteners Shown to Change How Body Processes Fat and Energy." Science Daily, Source: Experimental Biology 2018, April 23, 2018. https://www.sciencedaily.com/releases/2018/04/180423085440.htm...

Wilkerson, Jordan. "Why Roundup Ready Crops Have Lost Their Allure." University: The Graduate School of Arts and Sciences, Science in the News. Accessed January 19, 2019. http://sitn.hms..edu/flash/2015/roundup-ready-crops/.

Willis, Ally. "Shoppers and Brands Agree: We Want Proof It's Non-GMO!" Accessed March 11, 2020. https://livingnongmo.org/2020/03/09/shoppers-and-brands-agree-we-want-proof-its-non-gmo/

Wilson, Debra Rose. Healthline Editorial Team. "The Benefits of Vitamin D." November 13, 2017. https://www.healthline.com/health/food-nutrition/benefits-vitamin-d.

Wooley, Elizabeth. Richard N. Fogoros. "Top Fruit Choices for Diabetes Friendly Diets." Verywell Health.com. November 22, 2019. https://www.verywellhealth.com/my-top-5-best-fruits-for-diabetics-1087457.

Wootton-Beard PC, Brandt K, Fell D, Warner S, Ryan L. Effects of a beetroot juice with high neobetanin content on the early-phase insulin response in healthy volunteers. J Nutr Sci. 2014 Apr 30;3:e9. doi: 10.1017/jns.2014.7. PMID: 25191617; PMCID: PMC4153083. https://pubmed.ncbi.nlm.nih.gov/25191617/.

Younkin, Lainey. "Complete Keto Diet Food List: What You Can and Cannot Eat If You're on a Ketogenic Diet." Eatingwell.com. October 15, 2018. http://www.eatingwell.com/article/291245/complete-keto-diet-food-list-what-you-can-and-cannot-eat-if-youre-on-a-ketogenic-diet/.

"Xylitol: The Sweetener That Is Not So Sweet for Pets." ASPCA.org. The American Society for the Prevention of Cruelty to Animals® .September 20, 2019. https://www.aspca.org/news/xylitol-sweetener-not-so-sweet-pets.

Zeratsky, Katherine. "Is it Possible to Take Too Much Vitamin C?" Mayo Clinic. *Healthy Lifestyle: Nutrition and Healthy Eating.* Accessed May 27, 2020. https://www.mayoclinic.org/healthy-lifestyle/nutrition-and-healthy-eating/expert-answers/vitamin-c/faq-20058030.

Zeratsky, Katherine. "Which Type of Oil Should I Use for Cooking with High Heat?" Mayo Clinic. *Healthy Lifestyle: Nutrition and Healthy Eating.* Accessed December 2, 2020. https://www.mayoclinic.org/healthy-lifestyle/nutrition-and-healthy-eating/expert-answers/cooking-oil/faq-20058170.

Zimmer, Katarina. "How Toxic is the World's Most Popular Herbicide Roundup?" The Scientist. February 6, 2018. https://www.the-scientist.com/news-opinion/how-toxic-is-the-worlds-most-popular-herbicide-roundup-30308.

Made in the USA
Middletown, DE
20 October 2022